Adventure for everyone...

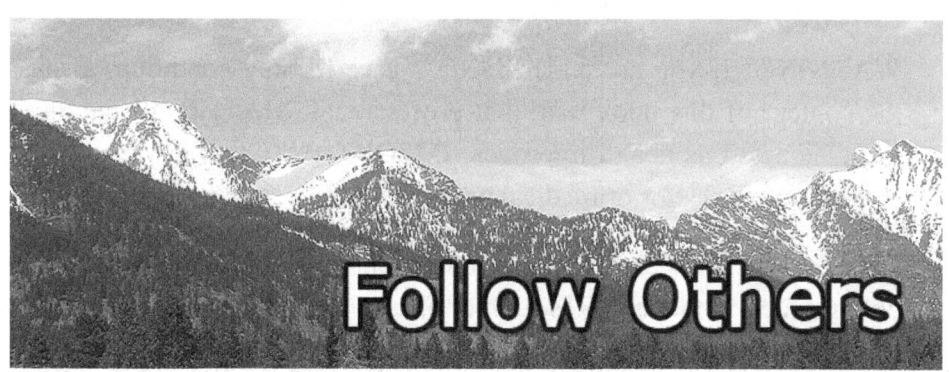

*Aging Wisdom from
Beatitudes, Nature, Kinfolk*

Donna A Ford

Follow Others: Aging Wisdom from Beatitudes, Nature, Kinfolk

Copyright © 2021 Donna A Ford

All rights reserved. No part of this book may be used or reproduced by any means, graphic, electronic, or mechanical, including photocopying, recording, taping or by any information storage retrieval system without the written permission of the author except in the case of brief quotations embodied in critical articles and reviews.

This book is a work of non-fiction. Unless otherwise noted, the author makes no explicit guarantees as to the accuracy of the information contained in this book and in some cases, names of people have been altered to protect their privacy.

WARNING: If you are under doctor's care for any condition, discuss the content of this book with that professional. Medications may need to be adjusted as health improves. IMPORTANT: It is always best to consult with a doctor or medical professional to get a proper diagnosis.

Trademark names of companies and their products are respected but not provided in the text. Research online.

Scripture taken from the King James Version of the Bible, unless otherwise indicated. Amplified New Testament as found in: The Layman's Parallel New Testament, published by Zondervan Publishing House © 1970.

Due to the dynamic nature of the Internet, any web addresses or links in this book may have changed since publication and no longer be valid.

ISBN: Print   978-1-7367331-1-0

          eBook   978-1-7367331-2-7

Print information available on the last page.

Follow Others: Aging Wisdom from Beatitudes, Nature, Kinfolk

Reviews

Karen Mains, Mainstay Ministries, Before We Go podcast. What a wonderful idea! Donna Ford has beautifully woven the Beatitudes throughout an approach to all aspects of the aging process. "Be happy..." "Be blessed..." this is a marvelous mediation tool for those of us among the elderly demographic. This look at becoming elders is comprehensive in its approach to the emotional, physical, psychological and spiritual aspects of the aging process. A job well done!

James Matthews, Technical Writer, retired. As a Baby Boomer in the silver years of my life, I've had to deal with many challenges. Physical changes, financial challenges, spiritual questioning. Ford describes her own journey through these obstacles and the journeys of those important people in her life, as guidance for the reader. The narrative is very thorough and can be identified with, all from the voice of a natural-born teacher. The asides about the Corliss family in Vermont are worth the price of admission on their own. Add to that the wide ranging health and exercise facts, tips and observations and the confirmation of spiritual values and support that brings, and Follow Others is a compelling read.

Rita LaRosa, Quality Manager. "Life is a wondrous adventure that needn't become routine just because of age."

Grace Thompson, Administrator, mental health office. The author masterfully weaves the truths of the Beatitudes into practical nutritional wisdom that she has learned over time. Aging doesn't have to be scary and intimidating, but we can garner years of experience from her and prepare ourselves to live the best life we can. Ford's handy nutrition guide makes it easy to look up a specific illness and quickly find applicable solutions. This is definitely a resource that will be well used for years to come.

Follow Others: Aging Wisdom from Beatitudes, Nature, Kinfolk

Acknowledgments

Thanks to all those who have lived through the several years of birthing this book. The prospective Christian agent who took the time to make important design suggestions and attempted to find a top-tier publisher willing to take on an unknown author. Volunteers among friends and relatives who read the two-hundred plus page volume in its early iterations and offered suggestions for making it better. Writer group members who pointed out the obvious grammatical errors. Facebook friends whose God-given words of encouragement kept me from giving up. Customers whose purchase and sharing helps preserve this wealth of information in one place for next generations.

Follow Others: Aging Wisdom from Beatitudes, Nature, Kinfolk

Introduction—Welcome Fellow Adventurer	1
Chapter 1—Aging Milestones	5
Part 1: Beatitudes	10
Chapter 2—Living Life Upside Down	11
Chapter 3—Leaving Legacy for Youth	27
Chapter 4—Living Apostles' Beatitudes	39
Chapter 5—Positive and Negative Relationships	47
Part 2: Nutrition	64
Chapter 6—To Your Good Health!	65
Chapter 7—External Aging is Universal	83
Chapter 8—Avoid Aging Diseases	113
Chapter 9—Aging By Gender	125
Part 3: Exercise	146
Chapter 10—Adventure Stirs the Bones	147
Chapter 11—Diet Fads and Fitness	161
Chapter 12—Motivation in Motion	181
Part 4: Life Changes	206
Chapter 13—Map Out Financial Plan	207
Chapter 14—Push To the Top	233
Afterword, About	249
Appendix A—Personal Health Defense	255
Resources	259
Indexes	265

Follow Others: Aging Wisdom from Beatitudes, Nature, Kinfolk

Dedication

I dedicate this story of my life's learning to my Vermont relatives, other family members and health and medical practitioners who helped me become the healthy, aging version of myself I am today.

Corliss Kinfolk. This story is inspired by my Vermont relatives, my guides to aging well. You will meet them later in this book.

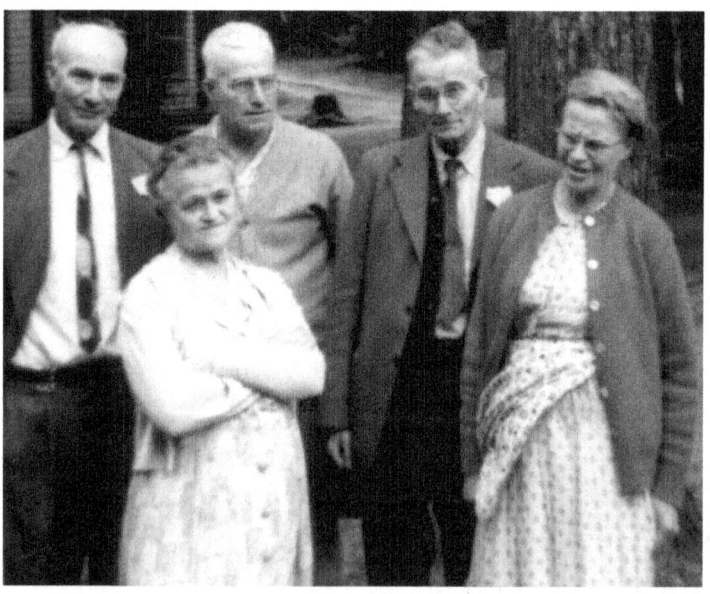

1965 – Picture taken at family reunion in their seventies.

Left to right, brothers: Valentine Corliss, Edwin Corliss, Harrison Corliss; Left to right, sisters: Flora Corliss Griffith (author's grandmother), Flossie Corliss Parker

My Corliss kinfolk knew how to make aging a true adventure!

Follow Others: Aging Wisdom from Beatitudes, Nature, Kinfolk

Introduction—Welcome Fellow Adventurer

"Wisdom is with the elderly, and understanding comes with long life." Job 12:12

Now is the time of life when young people may hold doors open for us based on looks. Doctors label us geriatric because of the age on file. As Jesus warned Peter, when we get old people will help put on our clothes and take us places we don't want to go. Can we forgive, overlook and keep going? The choice is yours—and mine.

Whether you have merely crossed the divide into middle age or are seeing your 50s and 60s in the rearview mirror, this book offers new ways of viewing the aging process. None is too old not to remember what it felt like to be a teen, the time when every life happening was a traumatic event.

Yet, somehow we survived. Now double those feelings of insecurity and sprinkle in hopelessness...our hair is thinning, our muscles are sagging, our belly is bulging, our neck looks like a turkey, our eyes aren't what they used to be! That's the typical view of aging.

Before anyone panics, this book and the success stories of others help to put things in perspective. Aging can enlarge our viewpoints, give us insight to spot fake news and provide the basis for evaluating latest medical claims and health creams. Just in case you are wondering if you need to read through this book, the shortened version below can make it simple to maintain health.

Three Ways to Build Health: Choose Two. Allowing for differences, we have been provided the choice of THREE ways to build health in

Follow Others: Aging Wisdom from Beatitudes, Nature, Kinfolk

the human body. And, it is not necessary to do all three immediately. However, you have to select at least TWO and pursue them diligently in order to live a long, full life on earth.

These health-building options are covered in Chapters found in Parts 1 through 3 of this book:

Part 1: Positive Thinking (based on the Beatitudes, not wishful thinking)

Part 2: Nutrition (more than just good food)

Part 3: Exercise (less than you think)

Part 4: Final chapters address financial planning and tough life choices whether married or single. Plus, within every chapter you will find bits of wisdom and inspiring family stories.

Changing Life Plans for Healthy Aging. The truth about aging is that most of us will live longer than projected and may have to adapt with separate plans for optimized life:

Plan for Fifties and Sixties—We have to change expectations and let youth be a memory. Focus on pursuing two of the three options for health: positive attitude; nutrition; exercise. Unfortunately we all know someone who threw their sixty-year-old hands in the air, and said, "What the heck!" A decade later that person, if still alive, may be dealing with doctors, drugs, unrelenting aches and pains or the big C.

Plan for Seventies onward—Only for the brave. Can we discover renewed energy and value for our lives while accepting some changes we dislike? We may realize the need for adding in that third option ignored in the first plan; for example, a fall may show the importance of exercise or an osteoporosis diagnosis reveals the need for improved nutrition.

Follow Others: Aging Wisdom from Beatitudes, Nature, Kinfolk

Pray or Call a Doctor? I wondered about this question in the days while my children were in grade school (they are in their 40s and 50s now). My conclusion then remains the same. Miraculous healing is similar to having quadruple bypass surgery. It can save us from immediate death. Unfortunately, if we return to our previous poor diet, lack of exercise, smoking habit and/or negative attitude, we could be in the same ICU within six months. Jesus told people he miraculously healed to "go and sin no more." Instead, you can pray for wisdom and guidance such as that I found and recorded in the pages of this book.

I am a great advocate for doctors because that was a career path I wanted to follow. The reason for admiration is because they have been trained in diagnosing sickness and disease. They may not have taken courses in nutrition, but diagnosis within their specialty is their expertise. They can tell you whether your toenail was damaged by stubbing or if it there is a melanoma cancer growing underneath. With a push of a toe, a young doctor can tell if a senior broke a femur in a fall before seeing any X-ray. My recommendation about dealing with health issues, is to go see your doctor and consider their recommendations. If like me, you cannot tolerate a pharmaceutical approach, then consult chapters in this book on generic aging and male/female issues. Perhaps you will discover a natural remedy solution, like Homeopathy, that works for you.

For those looking for health and healing wisdom, the information included in this book is not meant to supersede advice from a medical professional. The tips offered are generic and cannot possibly take into account your personal health information. However, they will provide you with key words to research and discuss with your doctor on current online topics.

Follow Others: Aging Wisdom from Beatitudes, Nature, Kinfolk

End Point: And you thought you had to wing Aging on your own!

Prayer Point: Let this book be the answer to someone's prayers.

Chapter 1—Aging Milestones

"So teach us to number our days that we may apply our hearts unto wisdom." Psalm 90:12

When God created the earth and committed it to the care of Adam and Eve, He instructed mankind to replenish the earth. A great-aunt saw a miracle of replenishment happen right in her own Vermont kitchen. And she was not the type to lie, or even exaggerate! Read about Aunt Flossie at the end of this chapter.

How many candles burned brightly on top of your last birthday cake? Or maybe you have called a moratorium on birthday celebrations. Whether you celebrate or not, our immediate world has pegged us into aging slots. This may begin with a mid-life event of some sort—perhaps an over-the-hill birthday party accompanied with black balloons. Hopefully it wasn't accompanied by a mid-life crisis. Here are some aging milestones including tales of my own.

Middle-Aged. This first label was innocently delivered by a fourteen-year-old when I was thirty-five. I made the mistake of asking him what he thought about my age (I was thinking about it!). His straight up answer was "middle-aged." Wisdom from the lips of our own offspring! Oops. Amazing how the ages of our children reflect on our milestones. (The youngest of my nine grandchildren just turned twenty-two as this book is readying for print! And there are nine great-grandchildren, too.)

Geriatric. The second label was delivered by a neurosurgeon. He had read the chart outside the room where I awaited a consult on neck issues. He entered the door, took one look and then kept his eyes

Follow Others: Aging Wisdom from Beatitudes, Nature, Kinfolk

down—literally for minutes. If he dared raise them, I could have read the label, Geriatric, that he expected to attach to every sixty-something female patient. He was embarrassed because of his prejudged assumption based on the record that did not equate with the woman before him. (I have aged well.)

Society Labels. We know about the Baby Boomers, Millennials and Generation Xers. Which label has society assigned to you? Many readers may fall into the same category as I do, baby boomer (or pre-boomer since born in 1944). With Dad in Europe fighting in World War II and Mom back in Vermont living with her parents, it was Grandfather that drove us in his model-T truck down the gravel road to the hospital where I was born. And if that bit of story doesn't age me, nothing can.

Millennials. A recent article said that this age group is one of the least healthy. Perhaps stressing about the environment and politics is bad for their health. If you have children in this age group consider sharing with them Chapters 2 through 5 about the Beatitudes and positive thinking.

The Family stories are about age-defying Vermont kinfolk. The Tips and Wisdom are short studies on nutritional or personality issues that I hope you consider fascinating and timely. These have strongly influenced me and will show up throughout this book. Such stories need extra space to tell properly. Additional Tips and Wisdom posts may appear on this blog based on reader and audience questions/feedback. http://donnaaford.com/blogs

Follow Others: Aging Wisdom from Beatitudes, Nature, Kinfolk

Turning Back Time Miracle. After turning fifty, I began to verbalize the obvious aging that appeared as a reflection in the mirror. A new wrinkle here; more grey hairs each week. But one day, God spoke from the Bible story about King Hezekiah's sun dial. Apparently God has a different view point about aging than family, doctors, society or we do. Here's the story and promise He gave me that day.

In the days when the Bible was written, the way one told the time of day was with a sundial. This device uses sun rays, that fall across a raised stationary indicator, to create a shadow pointing to the outer edge of the dial face. The dial has tick marks for each hour, similar to a non-digital (analog) watch. This Biblical story of a sundial occurred in 700 B.C. at the Jerusalem palace of King Hezekiah.

The king had been ill and expected to die. He was visited by God's prophet who delivered good news – Hezekiah would live another fifteen years. The 'anti-aging' remedy to be administered was a plaster of figs (sugar source still in use today) placed on top of the abscess.

How could Hezekiah be certain he would be healed? The prophet said God would move the shadow on the sundial ten degrees. Should He move it down ten degrees or back ten degrees? Hezekiah chose for it to move back ten degrees—that had never been seen before, a miracle.

Is this story a real event? If so, scientists should find ten degrees of time missing from the calculation of years. Guess what? They have found ten degrees plus 24 hours missing. If you want to know where the 24 hours went to, read the blog page: Joshua's twenty-four hour day.

Like King Hezekiah was promised fifteen more years, that discouraging mirror reflection seemed more and more to reverse—as miraculously as that sundial did. It wasn't until turning seventy that aging began to catch up with me again. A true story, I promise you.

Follow Others: Aging Wisdom from Beatitudes, Nature, Kinfolk

Aunt Flossie, Centenarian

Now meet the family member who to my knowledge lived the longest. Great Aunt Flossie lived into her 100th year. Some might have thought her to be "dour" but she was just a quiet New Englander.

Flossie provided care for her mother, my great-grandmother Achsa, during the last year of life until she passed away at 81. It was also Aunt Flossie who invited the preachers to her Vermont home for dinner in the following miracle story she told.

Aunt Flossie prayed earnestly for her sister Flora's ten children (including my mother) that they would all come to love the Lord Jesus. Prayers were partially answered in 1967 when my father and all six of us children were saved during a six-month period. Prayers for her nephews continued to be answered even as Flossie witnessed to them about the Lord when they visited her in the nursing home. She will assuredly meet these members of our family in heaven one day.

Flossie's Miracle Happened on Sunday. Preachers had driven up to Vermont from Connecticut and were now seated in her living room, right across the street from the little Gospel Hall where the Sunday service was held. While they chatted, Aunt Flossie was busy in the kitchen, just like a modern-day Martha. That's when she realized there was only one slab of butter left. In the 1950s and 60s, everyone served bread and butter at meal time. What could she do? If you blinked, you would drive through Woodbury, VT, and miss it. There was no store nearby to buy more butter. Besides, this was Sunday and stores were closed back then.

Of course, Flossie could have apologized in advance, saying something like, "That's all of the butter. Please use a little less." She insisted, a

Follow Others: Aging Wisdom from Beatitudes, Nature, Kinfolk

quarter century later, that she never said a word. In fact, native Vermonters seldom make useless remarks. Aunt Flossie did the only thing she knew to do. She prayed that there would be enough butter to last through the meal.

The guests pulled their chairs up to her table and gave thanks for the food spread before them. They passed heavy plates of food and then buttered their bread slices. They ate and talked. Every time Aunt Flossie glanced at the butter dish there was still more left—even after the guests, now full, pushed away from the table and thanked their hostess. When they left the house, she stood quietly in awe at having seen a miracle.

Here's hoping that the family stories in this book remind you of those who inspired you and shared their wisdom, which now helps to win at aging.

Part 1: Beatitudes

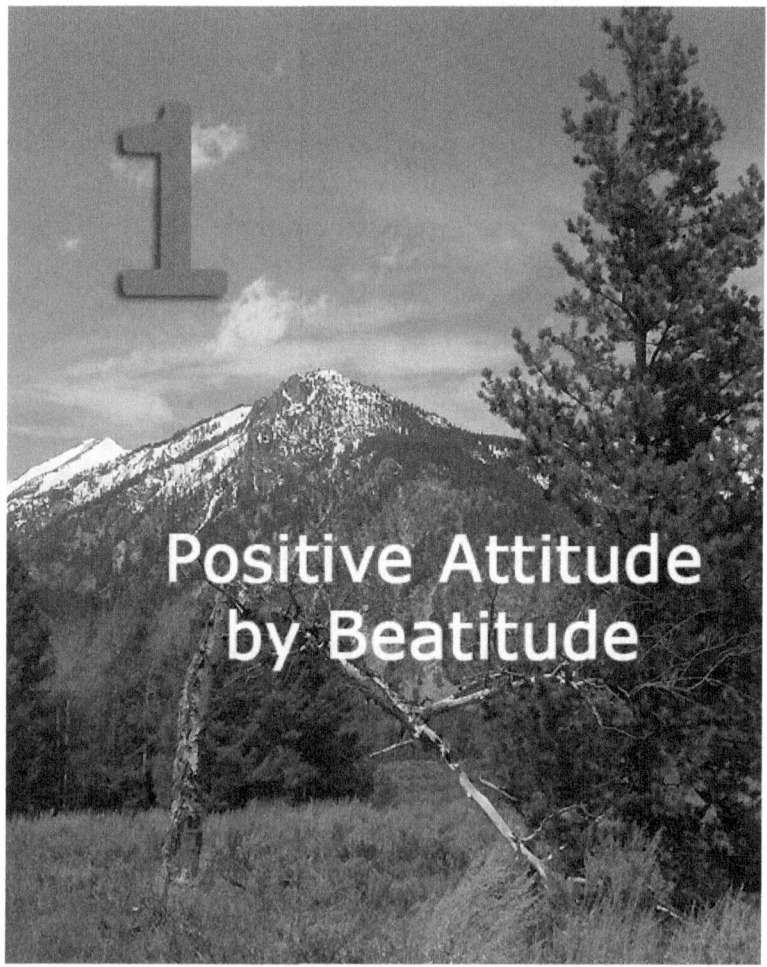

In This Part...

Chap2: Living Life Upside Down

Chap3: Leaving Legacy for Youth

Chap4: Living Apostles' Beatitudes

Chap5: Positive and Negative Relationships

Follow Others: Aging Wisdom from Beatitudes, Nature, Kinfolk

Beatitude: Blessed—happy, to be envied, and spiritually prosperous [that is, with life-joy and satisfaction in God's favor and salvation, regardless of their outward conditions]—are the poor in spirit (the humble, rating themselves insignificant), for theirs is the kingdom of heaven! Matthew 5:3 Amplified

Chapter 2—Living Life Upside Down

Grit reminds us of the western image of a cowboy equipped with his rope and known for his determination. He's the character played by Michael Landon in the "Little House on the Prairie" series, or the Lone Ranger and his Indian cohort, Tonto. He could be a she, the woman Jesus praised for the gift of her last pennies in the offering plate, or Mary who anointed Jesus for burial with the expensive box of ointment. I believe that is how Jesus saw the first beatitude played out, Grit minus the blaze of guns and saddles. Read Grit for Trials below.

Ours is the age when the Beatitudes that Jesus first taught his disciples finally make sense as rules for living well. We are the generation who understand the value of generational blessings. We live longer. We play videos on fat-burning diets and infomercials on air cookers. We avidly read magazine ads that tout the benefits of probiotics or yoga, willing to believe or at least hope to discover secrets of longevity.

Most exciting is brain research being done. Scientists promise that within our lifetime we can reprogram negative thoughts and add years to our lives. Jesus' beatitudes were way ahead of time on the subject of brain neuro plasticity!

The lack of interest people of Galilee had in the Beatitudes may relate to negative connotations of their day. Jewish hearers didn't want another set of tough laws to keep. Even Jesus' disciples showed so little

Follow Others: Aging Wisdom from Beatitudes, Nature, Kinfolk

enthusiasm that they never asked for an explanation, as they did regarding the parables.

The trick to understanding the Beatitudes is as simple as photography: use the negatives to create beautiful positives. That's what we will do throughout Chapters 2 and 3. And in Chapter 4 we will see how the Apostles chose to pass their own insights on to the church.

Consider this: In Jesus' time, Positive Thinking through the Beatitudes was the only anti-aging cure/remedy.

Beatitudes. Below is a list of the nine Beatitudes Jesus introduced to the crowd in his Sermon on the Mount. This list is quoted from the King James Version, Matthew 5: 3-12a. Other translations precede or end chapters throughout this book.

"Blessed are the poor in spirit: for theirs is the kingdom of heaven."

"Blessed are they that mourn: for they shall be comforted."

"Blessed are the meek: for they shall inherit the earth."

"Blessed are they which do hunger and thirst after righteousness: for they shall be filled."

"Blessed are the merciful: for they shall obtain mercy."

"Blessed are the pure in heart: for they shall see God."

"Blessed are the peacemakers: for they shall be called the children of God."

"Blessed are they which are persecuted for righteousness' sake: for theirs is the kingdom of heaven."

Follow Others: Aging Wisdom from Beatitudes, Nature, Kinfolk

"Blessed...when men shall revile you, and persecute you, and say all manner of evil against you falsely, for my sake. Rejoice and be exceeding glad for: great is your reward in heaven."

Each of these nine rules of God's kingdom on earth begins with the word, "Blessed." This can be translated "Very Happy" as well. How often does anyone who mourns immediately feel blessed? Ah, there's the key. While no one would feel happy at that moment, they might agree that happiness will return somehow, sometime. It did for a Bible character named Job, whose life you will read about in the next section.

What Jesus meant to extend with nine controversial rules announcing his new kingdom on earth was this blessing, or benefit as we'd say nowadays. Whenever our life is upside down, the best way to make sense of it is to view things upside down, too.

Centenarians Welcome to Apply. Everyone who lives past 90 is quizzed about what they think is the reason for their long life. Most of the time they claim it is something they eat or don't eat, do or don't do, married or single, etcetera. Here is a list of five traits necessary for a person to live a long life, 80, 90, even 100 plus years.

Grit

Courage

Enthusiasm

Confidence

Hope

Long life requires grit, hope, stamina, and most of all, protection from bad luck.

Follow Others: Aging Wisdom from Beatitudes, Nature, Kinfolk

Consider the Book of Job. In the Bible's Old Testament, there is a true character whose name was Job. The Book of Job is written as a Dramatic Poem. Job lived hundreds of years before the birth of Christ. He was not a relative (his name does not occur in either genealogy of the gospels), but he served as an example of a man who worshipped God and was protected from evil and not just because of his devotion. Job was mentioned by name for his good reputation both in the writings of the Old Testament by the prophet Ezekiel, and again in the New Testament by the Apostle James.

Job was favored by God throughout his life—until the day his faith was tested by disasters and suffering. Within a short span of time he lost his children, flocks, all his wealth and then his health. That's why to this day he is called "Poor Job".

I will let you in on a secret. Things turned around for Job, and he lived a happy and blessed life for 140 years after the events documented in this Old Testament story. Yes, Old Testament characters did live long lives.

Near the beginning of the book Job was indignant; he knew he did nothing amiss. Since he couldn't blame God without it being sin (he even told his wife not to do that), then who could he blame? Apparently, the presence of an adversary in the heavens was not well-known on earth at that time. Job may be the oldest book of the Bible.

What about our own time? Many ordinary people in the civilized western world believe that the devil is just a character at Halloween. Like Job, without an adversary who causes our troubles, God is the only one we can blame.

Let's take a deep look at five of the nine traits that Jesus promised would bring blessings, happiness and a long-life. The next covers the rest.

Follow Others: Aging Wisdom from Beatitudes, Nature, Kinfolk

Grit For Trials

"Blessed are the poor in spirit: for theirs is the kingdom of heaven." Matthew 5:3 KJV

Have you noticed poorer eyesight and hearing, lose of strength and memory? If you feel "poorly" in any of those areas the culprit is likely aging. And grit is the remedy to apply.

How does a person poor in spirit get Grit? I like the sound of this word, grit. It seems to come straight from a cowboy western where the good guys always win. Bible terms for this particular trait of longevity seem less attractive: endurance and long-suffering. Ugh! These imply 'hang on no matter what the consequences'; they never give in or give up, even if at the end of their rope, as the Message calls those who are poor in spirit. People full of potential, who hang in there until their personal world is righted.

Instead, consider the couch-potato—maybe you or me. If we always view ourselves on that faded cushion as watchers of other people who live exotic lives on TV, we can't see ourselves any other way. What might happen if we exercise a little—maybe stretch a hand or an arm? Jesus told a person with a withered hand to stretch it forth; guess what today's doctor would recommend—physical therapy to stretch the hand.

Joni Erikson Tada is a paraplegic who paints with a brush in her mouth, sings, has a radio talk show and sponsors camps and equipment drives to help other paraplegics and families. I recently met a woman who was friends with Joni as teens; they had planned to ride horses together the day after Joni was injured. Please note that Joni hasn't been cured of her disability, but she was healed of a poor spirit that would have kept her emotionally paralyzed forever. She has clung to the end of her rope since breaking her neck in a diving accident as a teen. Pure grit.

Follow Others: Aging Wisdom from Beatitudes, Nature, Kinfolk

How did Job trade his complaints for Grit? God listened in as he and his four friends analyzed Job's situation. Was he guilty of hidden sins: Job insisted not. Then maybe his children had sinned; Job had paid in advance with offerings on the altar. Did Job think he was greater than God? That was when the creator addressed Job. He asked whether Job had been there the moment after God spoke "Let there be Light," when the angels shouted with amazement as the dark curse on this earth was lifted. Was Job there when the animals of the sea and earth were created? Job began to see with new vision the wondrous God he had worshipped almost by rote. "Hitherto I spoke, but now I know."Grit had arrived and Job would heal when he prayed for his friends to see this new vision, too. The blessing he received was twice as many livestock (he was a cowboy after all) and a new family of descendents he would live long enough to tell about God's wonders.

Courage, not Fear

"Blessed are they which do hunger and thirst after righteousness: for they shall be filled." Matthew 5:6 KJV

Many have sought after the fountain of youth. What Jesus advised us to do instead was: Seek first the Kingdom. Whatever this means to you, courage is required to seek beyond what you think you are capable of. I have always admired people who are naturally courageous, almost as if they hunger and thirst for it.

My husband used to call me "Little Miss Much Afraid", after the main character of Hannah Hurd's book titled Mountains of Spices. And that was a fact and not an insult, believe me. I never smoked because I would have to hold a lighted match near my face. I was timid the first time I kissed my newborn son. I was afraid to get my ears pierced; at forty, I stood in line with a friend behind to give me courage. I whined out loud so much. When the young girl behind me got her ears pierced,

Follow Others: Aging Wisdom from Beatitudes, Nature, Kinfolk

her mother praised her as braver than that 'other woman'. And so forth. Enough stories to embarrass myself for the moment.

Christian speakers often tell their audience to "Do it afraid." I guess I can lay claim to at least that smidgeon of courage. How many petrified 40-year-old women would stand in line with children to get their ears pierced?

I wonder what other opportunities I have deprived myself of due to fear. David would never have become Israel's king if he cowered behind King Saul rather than charged toward Goliath. Paul wrote to his son-in-faith, Timothy: "God has not given us the spirit of fear (or aging for that matter, this author adds), but of power and love and of a sound mind." Who was afraid? Paul or Timothy? Both, since this was a dangerous time for early Christians.

Fear steals Courage. It takes a huge of amount of courage to face old age. That puts it bluntly—pure and simple. What does an avowed 'Little Miss Much Afraid' do at seventy-five as she inspects the wrinkles-in-time reflected in her mirror? Hint: she can't 'tesser' away like Madeleine L'Engle characters.

The reason we need courage is because, though aging, we still remember our youth. We take our stand in the bathroom as we stare at a foe stronger than Goliath. And all we have in our hands are some jars of cream and a handful of vitamins to do battle with.

Consider this: "The aging battle begins somewhere between the mirror and the mind."

What else did David take with him as he raced toward his enemy with a slingshot? He had three valuable things: the promises of God, previous experience when he resisted a bear and a lion, and the foolhardy bravery that comes with youth. OK, you know the song: two out of three aren't so bad. Let's consider our resources.

Follow Others: Aging Wisdom from Beatitudes, Nature, Kinfolk

If we commiserate with the mirrored image it clearly won't change things. Remembering the help we received in the past may at least provide a renewed perspective. The first framed Bible verse (Psalm 37) I was awarded for Sunday School attendance told me three times "Fret Not". Someone must have known my weakness. And I can't count how often I relied on God's help to train my children—with the expectation that He would keep the promise in Isaiah 54: 13 "All your children will be taught of the Lord and great will be the peace of your children." Without fail, even just five minutes before it was needed to prevent a sibling brawl or stubbornness, the right lesson was provided in words simple enough for me to teach and the children to understand. A PTL is called for right about here!

So Lord, how about a word for those of us aging visibly minute by minute, who still hunger and thirst for courage to do it well to your glory? The prophet Isaiah wrote the following promise of renewed youth centuries before Jesus was born. This pebble when shot with courage can defeat any old-age Goliath.

"Your youth is renewed like the Eagle's" Psalm 103:5b

The eagle makes its nest up on a perch—the highest that can be found. There is a myth circulating that at some point in the eagle's 30+ year life span, it plucks off its worn-out feathers and waits on that perch for renewal. Eagle specialists say this myth is not a true explanation of the Psalm. It may relate to the fact that the bald-headed eagle radically changes appearance over the first five years of life. Feathers on the head and neck change from gray to white. Beak color changes from black to yellow when fully grown.

Regardless of what the psalm refers to, both the verse and the beatitude encourage us to accept that we can never be twenty again. Then we can begin anew. Replace the false picture you see in that mirror with the image of a beautiful creature meant to soar the heights for an entire lifetime.

Follow Others: Aging Wisdom from Beatitudes, Nature, Kinfolk

And guys, this applies to you as well. We know you check that bald spot as often as we check our wrinkles-in-time. Let's all fly like the eagles with courage gained from God's promises.

Enthusiasm Glows

"Blessed are the pure in heart: for they shall see God." Matthew 5:8 KJV

What are the characteristics of someone who is pure in heart? I've labeled this enthusiasm because the literal translation of that word is "God within." Those filled with enthusiasm have not lost sight of the goal to reach the finish line. They are stripped down, single-minded and plan to run and win. They may be seniors who have downsized and invested their treasure in the next generation. They are the pure in heart.

Aglow with Enthusiasm. It has been said that eyes are the window of the soul. Eyes can mirror both happiness and misery, health and illness, surprise and fear, anger and peace, and of course, enthusiasm. Enthusiasm is so great that it escapes from more than the eyes. The whole body seems aglow, in a small way like the glory that surrounded Adam and Eve in the garden. And like the God who is the source of this spiritual glow, we feel the need to say something, do something and create something. That's why throughout the ages, each generation has developed unique ways to express their creativity: art forms (paint and sculpture, crafts and inventions), words (essays and poems, novels or history books) and songs with music. Musical instruments are mentioned as early as in the book of Genesis.

What makes great music? Like most people, you enjoy a favorite type of music and/or song. Did you ever consider what makes a piece memorable, draws generations to it? Would the shenanigans at

Woodstock have been a defining point of the 1960s without music from the greatest artists at that time?

As a writer, I think about creativity often. Where does it come from? Why do I have less than Stephen King or other novelists? Once I learned the definition of enthusiasm, my first thought was: why do I recognize great music even if it isn't my taste? The answer is that I recognize the genius behind the author/musician. I can hear their encounter with the mind of creator God. Perhaps through music we perceive the sounds of heaven reproduced as best a human being can achieve. Enthusiasm – God within.

Listen again to the music of your children and your great-grandchildren; if you strain you may be able to hear the greatness.

Confidence in Challenges

"Blessed are they that mourn: for they shall be comforted." Matthew 5:4 KJV

There is very little comfort to be found in 80 or 90 candles aflame atop a cake—no matter how lovingly it was made and iced with your name. This too might feel like a time to mourn—where did those years go, where have family members, friends gone? What happened to youth and dreams and jobs full of promise? Hopefully, you used them wisely—maybe most of the time if not always.

Losses that the aged mourn, followed by suggestions to keep going:

Spouse, family, friends – make new friends

Mentor, prayer warrior – your turn to step up to the plate

Youth – exercise; you shall run and not walk, even the youth stumble

Dreams – set new goals

Follow Others: Aging Wisdom from Beatitudes, Nature, Kinfolk

Job – volunteer, start business venture

You may challenge me on how to draw confidence out of this beatitude. I don't believe we can be comforted without confidence in the credibility of the One who promised it. When young we had to trust our parents. If at some point, our trust was misplaced, we switched to trusting only in ourselves. My mom vouched there was no Santa Claus, but my teacher said there was. Similarly, I cringe when someone says, "If you want something done right, do it yourself." They declare that their comfort rests in personal control alone.

How about tough things like a sun rise over the horizon every morning? And what does this person trust will keep oxygen levels right in the air we must breathe? Maybe that's why so many people worry about the environment nowadays. Their trust is in themselves.

A small child must trust in order to learn to walk. The more timid ones will not take a step unless they hold tight to someone's pinky finger or grip a large bag of potato chips. Poor things to put one's confidence in order to take that first step, ride a bicycle without training wheels or drive a car. Maybe this explains why I was always "little miss much afraid." I had little confidence and not much trust either.

What silly premises we accept as we age—that we might not make it to our next birthday, that the stairs are too steep or that this may be the last new car we buy. These predictions sap our strength and confidence. In my family story at the end of this chapter, you will meet a man who re-shingled a three-story roof at 72, but eight years later gave up life within two weeks of amputation of a leg. He had worked hard and devoted his all up to that point. What more might he have been able to accomplish for God in his 90th year? No one will ever know.

Sad if we mourn what we've lost, then lose the most valuable thing—our confidence, and give up.

"Find relief through grief." unknown

Follow Others: Aging Wisdom from Beatitudes, Nature, Kinfolk

Hope for Future—Victims or Victors

"Blessed are they which are persecuted for righteousness' sake: for theirs is the kingdom of heaven." Matthew 5:10 KJV

I consider this beatitude one of the scariest, but then we all know by now that I'm still "Little Miss Much Afraid." I've read stories of the horrors perpetrated on Christians by those Communists who adamantly refused to hear the gospel. In the 1970s atheists didn't want to believe it; they stopped those preaching so others couldn't either. There are current news stories of what relatives might do against a family member who accepts another religion. Sad stories also involve men in orange suits who knelt at the edge of water about to be beheaded.

John the Baptist—Messenger for God. Let's look at groups gathering beside waters in New Testament times. The Jewish people awaited their Messiah, someone political who would save them from the Romans. John the Baptist (so called because he urged people to repent and demonstrate this by water baptism) was not that Messiah—he confirmed this fact several times, declaring that he only came to point people toward the true Messiah. Today we would say he was Jesus' advanced marketing team whose appearance on the scene offered hope. For four hundred years there had been no prophets in Israel, and then came John.

I suspect John realized his end would not be good. The leaders were not interested in a Messiah who could cause trouble for them. However, the poor were interested, and they became more so when John declared Jesus to be the Lamb of God. This made John enemies in high places. Enemy number one was the ruler's wife. John told Herod he could not marry her because she had been the wife of Herod's brother. Just try to

Follow Others: Aging Wisdom from Beatitudes, Nature, Kinfolk

criticize anyone nowadays about who they decide to date or marry. Not a pretty sight.

When Herod's soldiers brought John into custody, Herodias came up with a plan. She instructed her teenage daughter to dance before the ruler and to make an outlandish request—John Baptist's head on a platter. Oh yes, that's not just a trite phrase; it was a fact in Bible times. Herodias' evil plan worked, but take one last look at what the beatitude promises. John advanced to God's kingdom, and Herodias' eternal fate was sealed as well.

Hope for the Aged. Let's take another look into that dreaded mirror. What do you see? Perhaps by now you remember that to view the world right you must see everything upside down. Have you noticed by now that the lines and wrinkles-in-time have smoothed, your youth is renewed like the eagle's, and hope is on your side as you believe the promises? If you are not quite sure yet, make it a habit to quote these verses out loud. Better yet memorize them so they sink done inside as grit and rise up to provoke confidence, while your eyes to glow with enthusiasm.

Uncle Ed, Church Builder

This is the story of my (great) Uncle Edwin Corliss who, with his wife, Nina, served the Gospel Hall in Hardwick, VT, for decades. There he helped build a small church, as local people attended Bible studies and meetings held by preachers who visited from out-of-state. Like Noah he is best remembered as a preacher of warnings and a builder for God, one who shaped me and my siblings into future church leaders who would persevere in his footsteps.

Follow Others: Aging Wisdom from Beatitudes, Nature, Kinfolk

I had heard about my great kinfolk most of my life. My Mom lived with them as a teenager in the 1930s. At that time Edwin and Nina lived in Hartford, CT, and worked at the Fuller Brush company. It was Aunt Nina's canary that saved my mother's life, literally. I always remember Aunt Nina owning a bird in an elaborate cage. At home alone one day, my mom noticed the bird had stopped singing. She went to check and the little creature was dead in the bottom of the cage. That was when Mom realized the gas jet was on in the kitchen and escaped outside before she too succumbed. That event spoke to her about eternity and she accepted what she had heard about salvation at the gospel hall.

I met Uncle Ed and Aunt Nina myself when they were in their 70s and 80s. I was young, not even mid-life yet. I didn't worry about aging, knew nothing about nutrition and health. But these kinfolk would inspire me to pursue my future bravely, adventurously. My siblings and I had accepted the Lord for ourselves. Now began four-hour treks north from Connecticut to Vermont to sit at their feet and imbibe of their years of spiritual wisdom. Ed was still preaching at the church.

For the first meeting with Uncle Ed, he stood high up on scaffolding he had erected beside the three-story church building. He was prepared to re-shingle its hip-style roof. At 72 this seemed a very old age to me not yet 30. Uncle Ed was not afraid of heights; when younger he worked in the Barre granite quarries.

I was in awe of him after that. Seems like I always looked up to him, like when he stepped up to the pulpit to preach, his teeth rattling from Parkinson's disease. His presence seemed almost spellbinding. Read the rest of Uncle Ed's story later in the book.

Follow Others: Aging Wisdom from Beatitudes, Nature, Kinfolk
End Point: *Maybe you didn't see these exact words, listed at the beginning of this chapter, in the Bible account of the Beatitudes. That is because of the changes that language undergoes over decades/centuries.

Prayer Point: God has not given us the spirit of fear [or spirit of aging even] but of power and love and of a sound mind. 2 Timothy 1:7

Follow Others: Aging Wisdom from Beatitudes, Nature, Kinfolk

Follow Others: Aging Wisdom from Beatitudes, Nature, Kinfolk

Beatitude: Blessed and enviably happy, [with a happiness produced by experience of God's favor and especially conditioned by the revelation of His matchless grace) are those who mourn, for they shall be comforted! Matthew 5:4 Amplified

Chapter 3—Leaving Legacy for Youth

Over forty years ago a wise preacher, Mervyn Paul, published a book with this catchy title, Lifetime is Training Time for Reigning Time. Like the Apostle Paul, Mervyn Paul realized that "All things that happen are for the good of those who love the Lord." That good may reveal itself on earth, in our lifetime or to the next generations. The lessons learned in trials—requiring us to be patient—these are gems that will adorn crowns awarded to us at Christ's judgment seat.

The day will come when the majority of people must leave middle-age behind to travel into the "land" of the aging. What do they pack in their bag as they approach that day? For some, the suitcase is heavy with fears about the future and its consequences. Others may decide to "wing it," pack nothing and take their chances—not wise considering that aging may take several decades or more to complete. Equally important to what they pack is what they leave behind for those who follow.

Although the immediate connotation seems to be financial, Jesus never said that you must leave your house debt-free to your children. Of course, it might make you both blessed. However, God knew ahead of time that the Romans would destroy all of Jerusalem and local property values would plummet.

Could a legacy be something as simple as that you taught your children how to cook well? Or that you researched the family genealogies? Do you inspire confidence and self-worth in young people? Did you teach

Follow Others: Aging Wisdom from Beatitudes, Nature, Kinfolk

them to love classical music and perhaps play an instrument? Fortunately, legacies of this nature are not just for your immediate family. Those who volunteer to be a Big Brother or Big Sister pass along blessings they received as children to those less fortunate. Near the end of this book, you can read about the simple legacy my Grandmother Flora and Uncle Jesse each left to ten children.

Children shouldn't have to look out for their parents; parents look out for the children." 2 Corinthians 12:14, the Message

Beatitudes to Pass On. Here is a list of four attributes/skills* that will turn any senior into a blessing to their family for the next three or four generations. No greater legacy could one leave to his or her children.

Be Content

Be Compassionate

Be Cooperative

Be Companion of Faithful Witnesses

*This list of traits completes the nine Beatitudes Jesus introduced to the crowd in his Sermon on the Mount. See previous list.

Personal Life Beatitude. My mother, Florence, raised her six children to follow one particular Beatitude. We had it quoted to us many a morning as we left to walk to school. And likely again when we arrived home grumbling in the afternoon. Her favorite beatitude simplification was: "Do unto others as you would have others do unto you." Luke 6:31. This is also known as the Golden Rule.

The words still stick to me like glue. Did someone mistreat me and am I tempted to pay them back? Do unto others... Should someone put an

Follow Others: Aging Wisdom from Beatitudes, Nature, Kinfolk

ice cube down my collar and not receive the same? Do unto others...once again. Still these eleven simple words repeat themselves, now in my seventies with my mother gone to her rest a decade before.

"Train up a child in the way he (or she) should go, and when he is old he will not depart from it." Proverbs 22:6

Be Content

"Blessed are the meek: for they shall inherit the earth." Matthew 5:5 KJV

No age group can beat the young with their ability to dream. Their dreams are not hampered by limitations, real or imagined. And their creative potential is off the charts. Then somewhere in their 30s, reality sets in. If the goal was to be a millionaire by 25, their twenties and thirties reveal that it did not happen. If they aged wisely, they will acknowledge setting the wrong goal. Only specific and measurable goals are achievable. Otherwise, they will blame themselves, others or God.

Retirees too can have reality issues. Loss of job title and work camaraderie can be especially stressful. I posted sticky notes with the words "Be Content" everywhere in our home while residing in New Hampshire. There, I lived a near-solitary life five days a week for seven years due to my husband's job and work schedule.

The Apostle Paul once said, "Godliness with contentment is great gain." He had learned to be content in whatever state of life he was in. Content in prison: yes. Content to meet kings: even then. Content as a son of a wealthy Roman Jew: yes. Content as a Christian stoned by Jewish brothers: even then.

Does that mean Paul gave up on his goals? Rather was that when he sought the Lord's plan for his life, not his own?

Follow Others: Aging Wisdom from Beatitudes, Nature, Kinfolk

I'm a hunter of gems and gold as well as a student of rocks and minerals in which they are found. I expect to be super pleased to see the gates, walls and streets of heaven—set with gems and paved with gold. Equally, I shall be pleased with any crown I might receive for being content. Read about "Lifetime is Training Time for Reigning Time" at the beginning of this chapter.

Be Compassionate

"Blessed are the merciful: for they shall obtain mercy." Matthew 5:7 KJV

The Old Testament has two compelling, short stories that demonstrate mercy or compassion. Each book is named after a woman: Esther and Ruth. Perhaps women tend to be more compassionate? Certainly, those who show compassion in life situations realize that they are put there for a purpose.

Esther—Came to the Kingdom for Such a Time. This young lady became a queen during the reign of the Medes and Persian. In her day, their laws were the final say and could not be altered. The previous queen had defied her husband by refusing to appear before his male companions. Her husband's angry words removed her from the office. The King's next word issued a command to round up the most beautiful maidens in his kingdom to vie for the Miss Universe crown, so to speak. And Esther, a Jew, was the winner.

Her Uncle Mordecai, told her never to mention her Jewish religion and she didn't. Until one day she had to take her chances because someone evil in the king's court sentenced her people to death and destruction. If she broke the law banning her from crossing into the King's court without permission, she could die immediately. To show compassion

Follow Others: Aging Wisdom from Beatitudes, Nature, Kinfolk

toward her people, she dared to accept the challenge made by her uncle—that she had come to the kingdom for such a time as this. You may know the outcome. Because of Esther's bravery, the Jewish people were permitted to fight against their enemies and the adversary in the King's court was executed.

Ruth—Drop Handfuls on Purpose. Another story of compassion happened in the time of the Judges and is written in the Book of Ruth. The story is about the arrival of Ruth and her mother-in-law, Naomi, returning from Moab. When Ruth's husband died in Moab, Naomi lost her last son.

Ruth chose to leave her homeland where people worshipped idols, to go with Naomi where the true God—as the Jewish people called the creator of heaven and earth—was worshipped. After these two ladies arrived in Bethlehem, Ruth went out into the grain fields to help with harvest. She and Naomi had returned poor, even though Naomi and her husband once lived in Bethlehem on family land. Miraculously it would seem, Ruth happened to reap grain on land that belonged to Boaz, a close relative of Naomi's family.

You can guess the outcome of this true romance: Boaz and Ruth were attracted to each other, even though he was older and she was a foreigner. Boaz advised his workers to leave handfuls of grain on purpose in the fields for her to glean. Next, with a little push from Naomi, Boaz offered to marry Ruth. Unless another family relative wanted to keep this ancient Jewish custom—marrying the wife of a deceased person to purchase their inheritance. This other relative passed on to Boaz the right to redeem the land. Boaz and Ruth married. Naomi became the nursemaid of their child, Obed, the future father of Jesse and grandfather of King David.

An extra display of compassion to note: Ruth, a Moabitess, was accepted into the Jewish birth lineage of Jesus as recorded in the

Follow Others: Aging Wisdom from Beatitudes, Nature, Kinfolk

Gospel of Matthew. Moabite men, however, were excluded from a Jewish congregation.

Be Cooperative

"Blessed are the peacemakers: for they shall be called the children of God." Matthew 5:9 KJV

Isn't it strange that we most often define a peacemaker in relation to an opposite: War.

Conscientious Objector. When Jesus pronounced blessings on those who make peace, did he mean conscientious objectors to war? Many religious groups refuse to serve their country as soldiers when drafted. They will accept noncombatant positions such as ambulance driver. The question remains: is refusal to fight the same as making peace?

Peace Keeper. In his book "Dancing in No Man's Land" published by NavPress, author Brian Jennings believes that a peace keeper is not neutral. In time of war, the peace keeper hunkers down in a bunker filled with people of like opinion. They remain close by the designated No Man's land, prepared to fight to enforce the status quo. Their goal is neither ending the warfare nor making peace.

Another definition - Harmony vs. Division. The black race believes music sounds best when they clap on beats 2 and 4; music of the white race seems better with claps on beats 1 and 3. If we humans would cooperate peacefully, what harmonious music we could make on every beat. There is someone who wants to divide us. If you think it is a Republican, you are wrong. If you blame the Democrats, wrong again.

When the issue concerns harmony within our circle, isn't "troublemaker" considered the opposite of peacemaker? The divider of

Follow Others: Aging Wisdom from Beatitudes, Nature, Kinfolk

people is the same troublemaker who entered the garden of Eden and had this face-to-face talk with Eve: What is it Adam told you? And what did God say? All lies, he claimed. "I know how to fix this mess; just follow my instructions and eat that damn fruit in spite of what God's rules are. You have rights, too."

In God's kingdom the troublemakers are not cooperative music makers.

Be Companion of Faithful Witnesses

"Blessed..when men shall revile you, and persecute you, and say all manner of evil against you falsely, for my sake. Rejoice and be exceeding glad for: great is your reward in heaven." Matthew 5:11, 12a KJV

Some things that Jesus said while here on earth, likewise true of his cousin John the Baptist, upset a lot of religious people. This last Beatitude is a 'hard saying' to understand. Most of us are looking for praise, not ridicule; rewards, not beheadings. So Jesus, how then are we supposed to rejoice and be exceeding glad? Not just a little glad—exceeding.

Ask the Christian martyrs. I never finished reading "Foxe's Book of Martyrs" because the book upset me too much. It tells the stories of early Christians who were tortured and martyred for their faith. They refused to deny what Jesus taught, including these Beatitudes which promised the coming of God's kingdom on earth. Corrupt political leaders of that day, including the Caesars of Rome, were not about to let the people of their realm practice any religion that claimed there was another King, Jesus.

What happens when two immovable opinions clash? In our day it means political mediation followed by war. For those who were taught to be peacemakers, the only recourse to avoid death was to disavow

Jesus and his kingdom on earth. They refused and that begins the history of the Roman coliseum games with its gory deaths and punishment of Christians as a warning to spectators.

What if Jesus' Kingdom had come immediately. Human history could have taken a different path. Without having to memorize the nine beatitudes, everyone's world view would have flipped over in an instant. Their eyes would have been opened and able to see from heaven's view point how to be blessed, happy and joyous.

But, it didn't go down that way, did it? Just like in the garden, Adam and Eve began to question everything and so did the people on the mount. In the garden God had clothed and sent mankind out to create their own world. Only God knew that he would send his son centuries later and make another offer of a kingdom on earth. The people in Jesus' day once again missed the opportunity. Still, God's son obediently went to the cross to die for the sins of all people.

You're right; none of this makes much sense— we inherited the world that refused God's kingdom. We might think we are compassionate, but with whom do we show mercy? Like the Pharisee, who knew that Moses' law stated he must love his neighbor, we too dare ask, "Who is my neighbor?"

Your Neighbor in the Kingdom. Jesus answered that question with the Good Samaritan parable (a story with a moral or teaching). He identified a certain Jew who fell prey to robbers on his travel between Jerusalem and Jericho. The robbers beat him, took his clothes and possessions and left him 'half-dead.' He must have cried out in pain because a Pharisee (religious Jewish teacher) walked slower but then hurried past. Next a Levite, who worked in the Jews temple, hurried by as well. They had important duties to perform.

Follow Others: Aging Wisdom from Beatitudes, Nature, Kinfolk

When a Samaritan passed that way, according to tradition he should have ignored the injured Jewish man. Samaritan's were disliked by the Jews. However, this Samaritan knew what compassion was like. He wrapped the man's wounds, clothed him in a garment and set him on the Samaritan's donkey. Then he brought the injured man to an inn and paid the housekeeper to take care of him.

The Samaritan received no reward at the time, but God noticed and he is promised a great reward in heaven. Likewise, to the early Christian martyrs burned at the stake, and to the conscientious objectors who went into battle fields without weapons of defense, God keeps accurate records of those who die in his service.

Val Corliss – Bulldozer Driver at 91

My (great) uncle Valentine Corliss was older than his brother Edwin, older and quieter. Uncle Ed did the preaching, but Uncle Val with his wife, Letha, cut their own firewood and sugared their own maple trees. Uncle Val was twenty years older than his wife. Aunt Letha still had strands of red hair that helped her woo the man, whom she preferred to call Tom. She was spunky and perhaps didn't think Valentine much of a name for her husband.

Though Uncle Val was quieter, his legacy was just as important to keeping the small church going. The Gospel Hall, which the five Corliss siblings started in 1943, required at least two male members in attendance. Their other brother, Harrison Corliss, didn't make it out to Sunday services very often. Most of those dear Corliss saints are now buried together in the South Woodbury Cemetery, on the hill that overlooks Woodbury Lake, Vermont. They await the rest of our family to meet them in Heaven.

Maple Sugar, Snow and Pickles. Have you ever tasted maple syrup drizzled on snow? Aunt Letha invited my parents, siblings and

Follow Others: Aging Wisdom from Beatitudes, Nature, Kinfolk

immediate family up their hill to taste it. Sweeeeet and that's why you needed a pickle to let the pucker reduce the sweet. Somehow she forgot to get donuts that are traditional for such a feast. She giggled and apologized while we stirred and stirred the syrup until creamy, when cold ice crystallized it into maple sugar. My first and only experience with maple syrup on snow is still memorable.

The Bulldozer and the Blizzard. I tell this story over and over because it impresses me even yet. No, it really wasn't a blizzard, although in a normal year in Vermont the snow banks are always at least four feet high. Now picture a narrow gravel road, still slick with fresh snow, that climbed steeply upward and around the final bend to Uncle Val's house. And picture a couple of foolish flat-landers, city folk who attempted to drive their small car loaded with four young kids up that hill to pay a Sunday visit. Next comes the bulldozer part.

My husband set the car's hand brake, got out and walked the last distance up around the corner to their farm. Lucky for us they were home. In a short time, Uncle Val sporting his usual plaid flannel shirt, rounded the bend atop his roaring bulldozer and proceeded to pull our car up the hill to his house. Don't you wonder what he thought about us young-folk on that hill in the middle of winter? I'll never know, though I can guess.

"When I am weak, then am I strong. Your strength is made perfect in weakness." 2nd Corinthians 12:10

Follow Others: Aging Wisdom from Beatitudes, Nature, Kinfolk

End Point: If you leave this chapter shaking your head wondering what Jesus wished to accomplish with his Beatitudes, you are not alone. On the day he preached his sermon on the mount, few understood. It seemed utter foolishness—even more so than the Laws of Moses. At least people were used to the ten commandments and the other law books of the Hebrews.

Jesus' disciples did not begin to understand these things fully until after his death, burial and resurrection. That is why Luke wrote down a simplified version of the Beatitudes as told to him by Mary or the apostles. To see Luke's version, read the Prayer Point at the end this chapter and those that follow.

Prayer Point: Beatitude according to Luke—Blessed be ye poor: for yours is the kingdom of God. Luke 6:20b KJV

Follow Others: Aging Wisdom from Beatitudes, Nature, Kinfolk

Follow Others: Aging Wisdom from Beatitudes, Nature, Kinfolk

Beatitude: Blessed—happy, blithesome, joyous, spiritually prosperous [that is, with life-joy and satisfaction in God's favor and salvation, regardless of their outward conditions]—are the meek (the mild, patient, long-suffering), for they will inherit the earth! Matthew 5:5 Amplified

Chapter 4—Living Apostles' Beatitudes

"..Staying alive to deliver your message, leave a legacy, complete your task." Unknown

Imagine yourself as one of Jesus twelve disciples. You spent every minute with him, doing his work for three years. You always expected him to become the ruler over an earthly kingdom. You studied his every move. Even asked him how to pray. And tried to live according to the rules of the Beatitudes. Then picture him taken away and crucified on a cross. You saw it all including the burial tomb.

The above is what Christianity claims happened to twelve ordinary men. And then on the third day Jesus rose again with a body that could walk through walls but still revealed nail prints in his hand. Now what? The men could return to fishing or previous trades.

But no, Jesus told them to wait for power; the Holy Spirit he promised would direct their paths as they spread the gospel to all nations. And that's what they did—became itinerant preachers to the people of the then-known world for the next thirty to forty years. While most of the Apostles would die early as martyrs, the four mentioned in this chapter lived long enough to call themselves "the Aged" or the "Elder".

What advice would you, as an aged Apostle, want to pass on to a church full of younger people? What would make it worth a lifetime of struggle? Why would these men keep serving even when tired and

Follow Others: Aging Wisdom from Beatitudes, Nature, Kinfolk

worn out? What would the future hold for the church once all those who knew Jesus personally were gone? Here are chunks and bits of advice they chose to offer the generations of Christians who would follow after them. You may spot some resemblance to the beatitudes.

Consider this: Beatitudes are the Psalms summarized; Epistles are the Beatitudes applied.

Advice from the Aged

We left the last chapter wondering what the disciples thought about the Beatitudes. Was it humanly possible to live by these rules of God's Kingdom? The church has indeed been built on the Apostles' legacy. America's constitution has proven that it is even possible to run a government by these rules—despite the obvious failings of mankind. Scattered throughout the rest of this book is advice from the Beatitudes as written by four who walked the earth during Jesus lifetime.

Paul: Good News. The Apostle Paul was once a serious student of the Old Testament, called Saul. (The New Testament was still future in his time). As a new Christian, Paul spent three years before he began to preach in the desert comparing Old Testament teachings and learning from the Holy Spirit about Jesus. Much of his writings explain the happenings of the gospels and Acts in light of Old Testament prophecies. After returning from his time of study in the desert, Paul certainly heard the other Apostles speak about the Beatitudes or rules for Jesus kingdom on earth.

Peter: Obedience. Peter was the leader of Jesus' band of disciples. He was the first one to preach the gospel to the Jews and also to the Gentiles (non-Jews). His input contributed to the gospel of Matthew.

While Paul described a rapture that could occur at any moment, it was Peter who later foretold of a day when there would be new heavens and

Follow Others: Aging Wisdom from Beatitudes, Nature, Kinfolk

a new earth. Both men wanted to encourage disciples and converts, offering hope that the persecution which followed Jesus death, burial and resurrection would not last indefinitely.

John : Christian Love. John who refers to himself in his gospel as the "disciple Jesus loved" is the author of four books in the New Testament. As predicted by Jesus, he was the only one of the twelve who died of old age. Exiled to an island offshore from Turkey for his faith, John wrote the book of Revelations. Three epistles were written after his release. Now feeling his age, he began the second and third letters, referring to himself as "The Elder."

James: Wisdom. The James who wrote this book was a half-brother to Jesus. He grew up in the home where Jesus was the eldest child and the moral leader among the siblings. Even Jesus' mother Mary told a servant at a wedding in Cana to do whatever Jesus said. What had been Jesus' focus as he grew up? The Beatitudes were an open proclamation of what Jesus practiced while living as a son in Joseph and Mary's home. The beatitudes also are a summary of the Old Testament Psalms, which Jesus is known to have memorized.

What Happened to All the Apostles?

This information is based on fact, circumstantial evidence and tradition. NOTE: None recanted their belief in Jesus' resurrection.

Simon/Peter—AD 64, Rome; crucified upside down

Andrew, brother of Peter—Date unknown, Achaia, southern Greece; crucified spread-eagled

James, son of Zebedee—AD 44, Jerusalem; beheaded by King Herod

John, brother of James—AD100, Ephesus; banished to Patmos, freed to die natural death

Follow Others: Aging Wisdom from Beatitudes, Nature, Kinfolk

Philip—Date unknown, Hierapolis, central Turkey; likely martyred

Bartholomew/Nathanael—Date unknown, Derbent, Caspian sea; flayed then beheaded

Thomas—Date unknown, Madras, India; speared to death

Matthew/Levi—Date unknown, Ethiopia or Persia; possibly martyred

James, son of Alphaeus—Date unknown, Egypt; martyred

Jude/Thaddaeus—Date unknown, Persia; killed with Simon Zealot

Simon Zealot—Date unknown, Persia; crucified or hacked to death

Judas Iscariot—Matthew 27: 3-10, Jerusalem; hung himself before Jesus died

Matthias—Date unknown, possibly Ethiopia; possibly martyred

Paul/ Saul of Tarsus—AD 64 or AD 37, Rome; beheaded

Power of Our Words

Jesus taught his disciples about the power of words. The apostles interpreted the Beatitudes and left their legacy for those who followed the Christian way. Modern preachers are teaching the same.

Reach for the Positive. At our house we remind each other to "not say anything we don't want to happen."

There is advice of all kinds out there nowadays. At least five people a day on social media send videos for you to watch and invitations to seminars that are guaranteed to extend your lifetime or at least make your final days more enjoyable. We can thank Norman Vincent Peale for introducing the world to Positive Thinking. And we can thank

Follow Others: Aging Wisdom from Beatitudes, Nature, Kinfolk

recent preachers for teaching disciples of Christ to speak prophecy over their own lives.

Preachers have put an emphasis on the power of our own words. Jesus' mother Mary told the wine servers to do whatever Jesus said. At some point in her life, she had come to rely on the power of Jesus to perform miracles—simply by obeying his words.

To age successfully we must control what we say to the mirror, the jokes on aging we laugh at and the way we see our future. What do you prophesy about yourself as a senior citizen of this world? Watch your words!

"I had a glimpse of the transformation that comes over people when you honor them as children of God." Norman Vincent Peale

Positive Thinking – Peale. Norman's parents were dedicated to their Christian values. This proved to be both a blessing and a hindrance to his spiritual growth. The excerpts below are from my "Miracle of the Call" book.

As a teen, Norman suffered from his own low self-confidence. As the young man and his father knelt in prayer, Norman acknowledged that he was giving his life to Jesus and letting go of all his inferiority feelings." A speech by William Jennings Bryant, made Norman even dare to consider becoming a public speaker himself.

Norman was still afflicted by low self-confidence when he arrived at Ohio Wesleyan College. So much so that his professor advised he read William James. James proposed that an inferiority complex was a combination of egotism and self-centeredness. Another widely-read author at Wesleyan was Ralph Waldo Emerson. Emersonian logic helped Peale understand that he was not alone in the conflicts he felt.

Follow Others: Aging Wisdom from Beatitudes, Nature, Kinfolk

Peale later would preach a practical Christianity inspired from Emerson's writings.

It is amazing that the person called to write the book—The Power of Positive Thinking—very much needed that power himself!

With a supportive wife, Norman Peale was free to focus on writing sermons and booklets, as well as his "Positive Thinking" book that stayed on a Best Seller chart for 186 weeks. He had found a way to present the Gospel so the average American, not educated in church terminology, could understand and accept it.

Prophet of your Own Life – Copeland. Kenneth Copeland believes that anything God wants done on earth must be spoken by a human being. Adam was responsible to name the animals; whatever he called them God agreed with that name. Adam prophesied that Eve would be the mother of all the living. Noah and Abraham were chosen to prophesy over the new earth after the flood, and again after Babel divided the earth.

Some times in the Bible a person's words were stopped due to unbelief. Those who built the tower of Babel had their words confounded. Families and family groups could understand each other but the multitude could no longer work together to build a tower to heaven. Their plan had been to never separate over the earth. Though the aged father of John the Baptist spoke words of doubt, he became silent until after his son's birth. Then he praised God and prophesized what would occur in the gospels.

Battlefield of the Mind. Joyce Meyer tried to keep from saying anything negative, after she realized that her words got her into trouble. This turned out to be impossible. That was when she began to speak out loud the things she wanted to happen. She wanted her books to sell and be read by others. She wanted people to attend her meetings. She wanted to help the poor of this world. Joyce began to change when she vocalized what she wanted to happen.

Follow Others: Aging Wisdom from Beatitudes, Nature, Kinfolk

Other people find it easier to hear God's voice for their life when they write or keep a journal. Read more in my blog post: Silent Miracle Retreat.

Family of Stone Masons

This chapter mentions the Apostles and modern preachers building up the church of Christ with words. Though they worked in stone, my relatives were good builders, too. I come from a family of stone cutters and masons. Wiry men with strength and skill to build that which they dreamed or others designed. They may have been a product of their times—stone masons bringing trade skills from Italy and Scotland to America were set to work in the early 20th century creating town halls, capital buildings and churches.

Granite Cutters in Vermont. They weren't afraid of hard work or heights. Scaffolding was rigged and climbed. That's where I first met one of my maternal great-uncles. Uncle Ed (everyone called him that) waved hello to me with one hand free and a hammer in the other. He was standing on the hip-style roof of the church building's third story. At seventy-two, he was semi-retired but still an able handyman. As a young man he worked at the Barre granite quarries—so would my grandfather, uncles and cousins. Uncle Ed lived to 80 and his wife Nina to 90.

Stone Masons from Italy in Connecticut. I grew up hearing the story of my paternal grandparents who crossed the ocean from Italy at the start of twentieth century to find work in Hartford, CT. While still in the old country, my grandfather, then thirty, contracted a job laying sidewalk with a well-to-do stone mason. When it came time to get paid for his labor, my grandfather asked to marry the lovely fifteen-year-old daughter in lieu of money. No dowry came with the wife though, so they had to move to America to earn a living laying stone. My Italian grandfather lived to be 84 in a tenement building in Hartford.

Follow Others: Aging Wisdom from Beatitudes, Nature, Kinfolk

End Point: "Wisdom is the ability to apply..knowledge." KCM Bible Note

That sums up the legacy left us by the Apostle James' writings. It also describes the legacy found within this book on nutrition and health. Anyone could purchase all of the books in my Resources list and come to similar conclusions. The miraculous part is that these books each arrived in my life in the sequence and timeframe when I needed to learn and apply their knowledge for myself and family. Amazingly, newer data has not contradicted what I learned in the 1970s. And new wisdom keeps arriving, now via social media.

Prayer Point: "When an elder dies, it's like a library has burned down." African proverb, from Saturday Evening Post Nov/Dec 2018

If you keep your wisdom within yourself, it dies with you. In a nutshell, that is my motivation to complete this book for my family and to benefit of others!

Follow Others: Aging Wisdom from Beatitudes, Nature, Kinfolk

Beatitude: Blessed and fortunate and happy and spiritually prosperous [that is, in the state where the born-again child of God enjoys His favor and salvation]—are those who hunger and thirst for righteousness (uprightness and right standing with God), for they shall be completely satisfied! Matthew 5:6 Amplified

Chapter 5—Positive and Negative Relationships

My daughter, Grace, and I became friends early on. We picked nosegays of wildflowers together on family walks on Vermont hillsides, while her three brothers ran on ahead. We girls were definitely outnumbered, even when we owned a female dog. There was no one else to giggle with over cups of hot cocoa on a cold winter night.

When Grace got pneumonia, she and I spent Christmas eve and the following day in the hospital. As an ornery four-year-old, she had refused to take the medicine prescribed for bronchitis, no matter how many ways I tried to hide it. Once we were home, I made it quite clear—if there ever was a next time she would have to go to the hospital alone, with no mom there to make sure the intravenous lines didn't hurt too much.

Now she has a daughter of her own, maybe more opinionated than she was. I'm sure some day she'll write a letter like this about her Abigail. I bet they'll be best friends, too."

True! And they are the 5th and 6th Amelias in my family tree. Read story of Grandma Flora in Chapter 11.

Follow Others: Aging Wisdom from Beatitudes, Nature, Kinfolk

Positive Relations

Family, friendships and sexual relationships are among our most precious human experiences. I recently found the above piece of prose on friendship—written when I was in my fifties, stored on an "ancient" hard drive, and luckily backed up to CD. It reminds me of the legacy we humans pass on to the next generations.

Family Share Much in Common; Friends Need Not. I was struck with the first line, which I purposely left out of the story above. I had written: Friends need not be the same age. And they can be related.

This reminded me that there are rules about friendships, especially when the friends are different from each other. We learn about these somewhere in our lifetime, either the hard way or intuitively. I list several of the rules of friendship below.

Friendship Rules by Age. People who are alike and the same age can grow bored with their friendship. That happened to me in high school. A best friend and I needed a year's sabbatical before we were friends again. Perhaps, we needed space to grow separately? And how true for families where younger members often need to mature before they are able to understand their parents.

People who are alike but were born in different decades will already be independent enough to enjoy minor differences. My spouse loves early songs of the seventies; now I know most words to those classics, too. He had to inform me about the Ohio Kent State shootings because I had been a busy mother at that time in my life. Nine years difference seems to energize, rather than divide our friendship.

Follow Others: Aging Wisdom from Beatitudes, Nature, Kinfolk

Friendship Rules by Gender. Who taught us how to bond? It seems to be inherent to our gender.

Male friendships center around shared activities. Males bond while underneath cars or in front of a TV football game. They prefer to sit on stools beside each other passing bottles of beer.

Female friendships revolve around shared experience or taste in fashion and decor. They support and encourage one another and wish to look at their female friend across a table over lunch or tea.

Male and female friendships stumble due to such simple differences, including this one rule. When a female talks about a problem, the male thinks he should solve it. A female friend would know to listen instead.

Friendship Rules about Race. The unspoken rules for interracial friendships appear to grow more complicated every day. We tip-toe around one another in the attempt not to offend. In the age and gender rules above, there is room for variables. In racial friendships there is only one clear rule: both parties must agree to toss out all acquired barriers for the sake of the relationship.

That is why racial friendships often occur at work or in romance—where the need for the friendship provides enough motivation to focus on shared values. Friendships matter.

Friendship Rules about Pets. I wasn't born with the Pet-gene; but so many people are. A pet can reduce stress and lower blood pressure. Even then there are rules. The human must be perceived as the Alpha party in the friendship. Otherwise, the pet will own you, not vice versa. Pet training is about how to behave in a pack relationship.

Follow Others: Aging Wisdom from Beatitudes, Nature, Kinfolk

Friendship Rules about Singles and Married Friends.

Mistakes that married friends make regarding single friends: Play match maker; Accept repeat "No" answers without challenging; Forget to include singles in group gatherings

Goofs single friends make: Mistake friendliness for pity; Allow inertia to take over

Friendships are a Luxury, not Necessity. Certain personality styles make it difficult to find friendships. My style, for instance, wants only to discuss subjects of immense significance. Only someone with a similar personality style can appreciate these topics along with me.

Once every few decades, I meet someone who shares my interests. The joy experienced immediately between us is one of intense understanding. I never want to give this up. Unfortunately, time passes and we each move on to another job, another location, another assignment to be a friend. When the inevitable happens, this quote, found ages ago, becomes my strength. How much pain those simple words eliminate!

"Having someone understand you is a luxury." Then I add, "...that means it is not a necessity."

The special need of singles to have friendships must be noted here. Family, such as grandchildren, even former spouses and their family, may be the best sources for finding friends. Membership in clubs and church groups are good sources too, but being house-ridden complicates that option.

Follow Others: Aging Wisdom from Beatitudes, Nature, Kinfolk

Lucky is any person who has a lifetime friend, but aging can remove even these. Look forward to having many new friends enter your life, no matter for how short a time or how old you each are.

Friends As A Mirror. A recent Bible story I read also illustrates the rarity of true friendships. The souls of Jonathan and David were knit together by the unique relationship they shared through King Saul. 1 Samuel 18:1. King Saul wanted his son Jonathan to become king after Saul died. He knew that if David lived, Jonathan did not stand a chance to be king. So Saul tried repeatedly to kill David.

Lesser men than Jonathan and David might have become mortal enemies. Instead they both achieved greatness in their lives through their friendship. The writer of a daily devotional, Shane Johnson, stated that true friends find the "mirror" of their souls and say with awe, "What you too" understand me?

Intimate Relationships in Aging

Life Partners. At some point in our lives death begins to separate life partners. Since the usual cause is health-related issues, it behooves us to encourage our spouses to eat well, exercise and stay positive about aging. I remind my spouse how many dollars a month I spend on the food supplements I lovingly put in a daily pill holder for him. Thankfully, he is willing to take them.

Is there sexual attraction after aging? Can we find a mate that we can enjoy sex with into our seventies? On TV, they advertise websites that match singles over 50 years of age. For example, www.ourtime.com. A recent Mayo Clinic newsletter suggested intimate positions that would be comfortable to partner(s) who had various orthopedic surgeries.

Follow Others: Aging Wisdom from Beatitudes, Nature, Kinfolk

Second Chances at Love. Consider some obstacles that can thwart beginning a romantic relationship later in life. Remember, there are really no exact rules to fit all cases.

Marriage Options: What does the church say? Previous partner alive? Prenuptial needed? Adult children to consider?

Financial: Obligations determine whether a relationship can prove successful. Two homes—which one to live in or sell? Debts owned by one—will the other help pay them off?

Religious Options: Which church or religion to attend? Burial with which spouse?

Physical Limitations—See chapter 9 for Gender-specific health issues.

Caregiver for Family Member. The decision to care for an elderly parent at home is fraught with emotional issues resulting from role reversal. Often, the first consideration is the needs of the elderly and the second is financial. Few sons or daughters consider the enormous benefits there can be for the caregiver.

I recently read a small memoir titled, Present Bouquets, which tells the daughter's story of moving home with her elderly mother who lived into her nineties.

Benefits of having a family member as caregiver: Re-acquaint with childhood places and friends; Resolve grudges and/or misunderstandings; Praise parent for all they accomplished; Allow the elderly to do for themselves, and provide options when no longer possible; Listen to the shared family stories, the telling of which keeps the elder's mind sharp

Follow Others: Aging Wisdom from Beatitudes, Nature, Kinfolk

Never Too Late to Master Communication. Over the years I learned a great deal about relationships and communication styles. The information below came along at a timely point in my life.

A teacher of middle school students wondered why it seemed impossible to teach specific students. These wiggled and jiggled or ran around the room. Her book published originally in 1991 about their inability to communicate well was called, The Art of the Possible.

Markova's research developed a theory on how the brain processes information. She divided the tasks of a brain into three phases: Do, Think and Feel. According to Markova, information flows through the brain inward from the Do phase to the Think phase, circles around at the Feel phase and returns outward to the start point.

You've probably heard of visual or audio learners. The fact is that everyone's brain uses a combination of all three—audio, visual and kinesthetic responses. The problem with communication results from the fact that Kinesthetic has little ability to communicate. It can nod, it can wiggle, it can walk, but it can't communicate by the methods favored in our society: it can't write or talk. It processes information received from the other senses: touch, temperature, etc. Other phases interpret for silent Kinesthetic.

How we get along with our spouse, children, parents or boss depends of how each person is wired to communicate best. Here are possible combinations:

Both persons have one response type in common; workable.

Two persons have the exact opposite communication style; workable over time.

Neither person has a response type in common; poor communicators, need third person.

Follow Others: Aging Wisdom from Beatitudes, Nature, Kinfolk

Two persons have exactly the same communication style; ideal.

Communication strategies also apply to interaction with children, in-laws and parents. There are work-a-rounds, of course, unknowingly practiced by a person who wants to resolve their own silent kinesthetic bottle-neck.

At work it is equally important that we know how to communicate well with our boss and our peers. Based on their Think-phase, some want written memos; others need to discuss. We can discover the best job for ourselves, based on our Do-phase.

Leave a written or verbal legacy based on when your Visual or Audio processing works best:

Visual Doer types: write a memoir in the morning

Visual Thinker types: write a memoir or journal in a diary afternoon or evening

Audio Doer types: record a CD, DVD or podcast in the morning

Read my Silent Retreat Miracle blog post that explains this at: https://miraclecalls.wordpress.com/2016/03/11/silent-retreat-miracle/

Negative Relations

Witnessing in the Workspace. I've already hinted at the trouble in relationships that can be caused by Political Correctness at work. The Apostles learned that people would listen when they demonstrate the love that Jesus said identifies us as His followers. No one verbally objected if I said "thank God that you weren't hurt" after they told of some trouble. But their eyes said what they really believed. Did they look away? Did they agree, "Yes, thank God." Did they seem to want to talk? Loving of people gives us the right to mention God even in the work place.

Political Correctness. Through research, I discovered a 'gem' of a thought about what's the same and what's different after two major events turned life on this planet upside-down.

Faith in the Workspace – Focus on What's the Same

What's changed since 9-11?—God is IN; Jesus is politically incorrect; People are uncertain.

What's the same for Christians?—Our personality, temperament, life experience; Our Co-mission.

What changed between Passover and Pentecost?—Jesus was resurrected; the Word was explained; the Holy Spirit came down.

What was the same for disciples?—The disciples' personality, temperament, life experience; They had been with Jesus.

Resist the Negative. Like Eve in the garden of Eden, we are tempted to react and think negatively. We doubt that the God of the Universe is loving. We think we must fix issues ourselves. Here are true stories about a few far-fetched ideas we may imbibe.

Love my Enemy – Is that even possible? At one time it was fun to write out the shopping list to feeding 75 people over two days. I liked to cook at our church's annual conference. That day, however, it felt like a huge chore. My great uncles and aunts had kept the small church active since the 1940s. In the early 1970s my parents and teenage siblings, along with my husband and our four lively children moved up north to help out. I helped fill the generation gap that existed in the church. And it proved to be a lot of responsibility.

If I knew the term "burn out", I would have understood. At that moment I only knew to ask the Lord for help. To please send along someone to take over the responsibilities I felt dragging me down. My replacement soon arrived, but things did not go well between us. While that earlier prayer helped remove the sting of words, the tension at church grew. Somewhere, I can't remember the exact point, I became aware that all my admiration had turned to hate. I had acquired an enemy, and all the logic I tried to wield could not change either her opinion of me or my emotional response.

Is it possible to hate someone who is an answer to prayer? It is for a fact. Later, I would learn that one must love, or at least admire, a person first in order to hate them. That knowledge paved the way for forgiveness to occur and cleansed my mind of all remembered offenses.

Root of Bitterness / Offenses. In my lifetime I have seen many walls built up in society based exclusively on bitterness. Even Adam and Eve blamed others.

In America since the 1800s, the red man has had every reason to resent the white man for taking his land.

More recently, the immergence of L.G.B.T.Q. groups encourages bitter feelings against heterosexuals. Fear is purported as a motive, but political clout seems pretty important as well.

Racism and BLM pits blacks against whites. Wait, that sounds almost like a dog-fight! Each side is certain they are not responsible, nor guilty. It sounds more like how Adam blamed Eve and she blamed the serpent.

Follow Others: Aging Wisdom from Beatitudes, Nature, Kinfolk

How about the Me-Too groups forming around victimhood. Has the feminist movement enlarged the divide that already existed between men and women?

Immigrants from poorer countries feel they have the right to march over the border and apply for Social Security. Tax payers believe they don't.

It's not that walls didn't exist in earlier times. Ancient Chinese and Welsh walls are evidence of that. Rather it is that now the walls are seen as a badge of honor. What about the soldiers who fought and laid down their lives for all Americans? They saved fellow soldiers of a different color or nationality in order to protect freedom. They deserve a badge of honor rather than cases of PTSD.

Victimhood. The bad thing about victims is that there must also be a bully. I'm on record now that I dislike both words, victim and bully—immensely. They give people license to practice self-pity, expect sympathy or show hatred. These are all negative feelings. Consider Jesus' response on the cross.

Jesus had became a victim of Jewish politics, it would seem. He knew better—that He was born a son here on earth to obediently do the will of the Father. The Father's will included his hand-over by Jewish leaders to be beaten and then sacrificed for sinners on a Roman cross.

Jesus could have blamed Judas for betrayal of their friendship. He could have blamed the Jewish leaders of greed and condemned their actions. He could have hated the Roman ruler who ordered him to be whipped and then crucified, or cursed the soldiers who bargained for his clothes and made him drink vinegar instead of wine.

But He had delivered the Beatitudes, those upside-down rules for his Kingdom on earth. So what did he say rather? "Father forgive them for they know not what they do." Oh, they knew how to work the system and get rid of a troublemaker. What they didn't know was that they actually ordered the death of their Creator and condemned themselves.

Jesus said: "Father forgive them for they know not what they do." Luke 23:34

Avoid Depression and Anxiety. These twin offenders can negatively affect the brain chemistry of an individual. Poor nutrition and stress are major contributors to these disruptions. Loss of a spouse or health setbacks are serious stressors for seniors. Even the minor stress of low sun-levels in northern winters, is known to cause seasonal affective disorder (SAD) depression. And once experienced, the body and mind seem to trigger preparation for the return of symptoms—a self-fulfilling prophecy.

You should research: Herbs, oils and techniques that calm; Hot baths and saunas; Serotonin stimulators including exercise; Seek to be content.

Depression, Resentment and Self-Pity. Depression can settle over anyone at certain moments in life. Examples might be: when a sibling achieves or receives a success that you wanted; when a friend takes a cruise or travels overseas to place(s) you always wanted to visit; when others spread lies about you; or a promotion passes you by.

To rule out brain chemistry issues, this type of depression needs to be professionally addressed before it proceeds to chronic depression. Talk to a Christian friend or counselor. Or simply tell God honestly how you feel, because He already knows. The solution is simple, but self-examination is tough.

Follow Others: Aging Wisdom from Beatitudes, Nature, Kinfolk

Here is a simple formula I learned from a Christian book and memorized decades ago. The author, whose name I have forgotten, wrote the solution as an equation:

Resentment x Self-pity = Depression

I've occasionally given in to self-pity—so and so did or didn't do whatever. I've become resentful that I had to remain while another went—seldom vice versa because I like to travel. Those warm and righteous feelings settle in deep down and equal an unavoidable case of depression. Luckily for me, I hate depression more than I like feeling righteous. My mom was admittedly depressed from a teen onwards, but my dad was an extrovert. I wanted nothing to do with depression— EVER. Should I catch this scourge creeping anywhere near my mind, I 'fess up to my nasty feelings as I peel them away, one by one, like blankets that cover and justify my hurts. Didn't I deserve..? No. Why did they..? Not your concern. Follow me, Jesus has said. And the depressive spirit has lifted out of my mind.

"You can be pitiful or powerful, but you can't be both." Joyce Meyers

Break Habits and Addictions. Brain researchers have discovered how thoughts are created. More excitedly, according to researcher Dr. Caroline Leaf, is the fact that thoughts can be changed. When the Bible says to think on those things...whatsoever is pure and lovely**, it hints that thoughts can be altered by attaching a positive emotion to the thought.

Dr. Leaf describes an individual thought as resembling a tree. The more time we spend thinking about it, branch-like attachments can grow or shrink. This ability to change thought is called neuro plasticity. Researchers say it takes four days to change the emotional pathway between a thought and an attached emotion. If the thought is positive, the brain fills with a positive chemical that could be called Love. If the thought is negative, the brain experiences a chemical cloud that appears to be the opposite of Love.

A habit is the addiction to a particular way of considering a specific thought. A new habit can be created within 21 days. Using Dr. Leaf's 5-step process of revisiting an existing thought from a positive viewpoint, new emotional pathways can form. The sooner we respond against the introduction of a negative thought, the better.

One popular comedian told in her biography that when alcohol was disrupting her childhood home she wondered where God was. One day she realized He had been with her the whole time. That realization produced a new emotion which allowed her to forgive family members.

As a woman and founder of the American Red Cross, Clara Barton had many vocal enemies. When a staff member mentioned a particularly disagreeable scenario involving one of those enemies, Barton claimed that she "distinctly remembered forgetting" it. Neuro plasticity could have made that statement possible and true.

**The Apostle Paul left this message for the Christians at the city of Phillipi, and for those of us who would come later.

Think on These Things

"Finally, brethren, whatsoever things are: true, honest, just, pure, lovely, of good report; if there be any virtue, and if there be any praise, think on these things." (Philippians 4:8)

Follow Others: Aging Wisdom from Beatitudes, Nature, Kinfolk

Staying Healthy Chases Negativity

As I write this section it is winter in the Northern Hemisphere. Women are susceptible to feeling depressed due to the effect lower levels of sunshine have on their hormones. This is common enough to have a name: Seasonal Affective Disorder (SAD) and solution, special lighting that simulates sunshine.

Like handling negative thoughts, the sooner you respond to symptoms of illness or disease, the less apt it is to manifest with full-blown fury in your body. The complete article to be found in Appendix A provides proven rapid responses I have used for resisting these common illnesses: Colds; Flu; Shingles; Nausea, Vomiting, and Diarrhea

The desired response time is within 20-30 minutes after the first symptom. This might be announced by a headache, cough, sore throat or general malaise. It may be passed on from another sick person, come on due to planning for travel or event, following stress—whatever causes your resistance to be lower than normal.

Because the most effective healing response time is less than one hour, homeopathic remedies are the quickest and least disruptive choices for your body. Homeopathic remedies can be delivered sub-lingual (under the tongue), in sugar pills or alcohol tinctures in water for adults. The suggested remedies in this chapter are proven to work universally or ones that I personally have found effective. A second round of remedies, herbal and/or OTC can be added as needed.

WARNING: If you try any remedy listed in Appendix A, be aware that a delay to see a doctor could prevent diagnosis and timely intervention for serious issues!

Follow Others: Aging Wisdom from Beatitudes, Nature, Kinfolk

Edna and Forgiveness

She was a pillar of the local church where my great-uncles and aunts worshipped. We rented her large house after she moved into a small trailer. Edna was the aunt of my uncle's wife. And she was an example of Christianity lived out.

When we rented that house, Edna's nephew came by to offer his roof-cleaning services. In Vermont this help is almost mandatory, but especially that year when snowfall exceeded 100-year records. Home with three small children, I was sociable on his visits and talked to him about the Lord. Apparently, this upset him a bit more than he let on.

One day the milk delivery man missed our house. Three children younger than four years without milk could be disastrous. My husband had the car and worked at a bank one hour's drive away. I called the milk providers to find out what happened and was told that a woman called and cancelled the delivery. Oh, my, did I put on my protective, mother-bear personality immediately!

The only ones who knew about the milk delivery were Edna and her nephew. The next day was a weekend. My husband and I went over to confront Edna, since it was a woman who had cancelled the delivery. I can still see the raised donuts like balloons rising on her countertop as we insinuated and then apologized profusely. We never did figure out for sure, but apparently the nephew got someone to call and cancel. Edna was innocent. And more than that she was forgiving. I'll never forget her graciousness—so like God's.

Follow Others: Aging Wisdom from Beatitudes, Nature, Kinfolk

End Point: As an introvert, I was fearful and apt to avoid making friendships. Once I learned why we behave differently than others, my fears vanished and I could begin to enjoy the people who came into my life. You may want to investigate some of the books in the Resources list under the category of Personality/brain/inspiration.

I would love to hear that something you learned within these first chapters has been of help to you. Please contact me: author@donnaaford.com

Prayer Point: Beatitude according to Luke—Blessed are ye that hunger now: for ye shall be filled. Luke 6:21a

Part 2: Nutrition

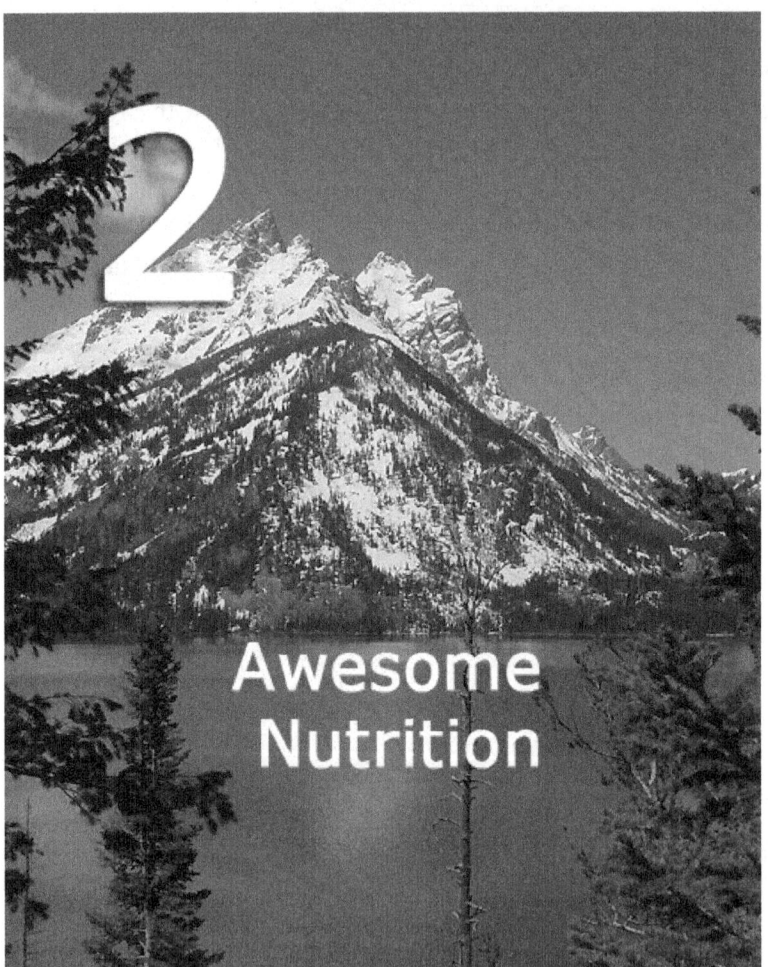

In this Part...

Chap6: To Your Good Health

Chap7: External Aging is Universal

Chap8: Avoid Aging Diseases

Chap9: Aging By Gender

Follow Others: Aging Wisdom from Beatitudes, Nature, Kinfolk

Beatitude: Blessed—happy, to be envied, and spiritually prosperous [that is, with life-joy and satisfaction in God's favor and salvation, regardless of their outward conditions]—are the merciful, for they shall obtain mercy! Matthew 5:7 Amplified

Chapter 6—To Your Good Health!

"We hang the very heavy weight of our happiness on the very thin wire of our health." Charles Swindoll

If I had to pick only two supplements to take for the remainder of my life, I would probably choose these two powerful youth restorers: CoQ10 and L-Carnitine. Mind you I take a LOT of vitamins and supplements. Then what is so special about these two? Read Youth Restorers section.

Aging ain't fun—unless we can manage to do it while in good health. This means that not only do we need to change our attitude about aging as suggested in earlier chapters, we must also optimize our health for the aging adventure ahead.

You Can Outlive Expectations. You Can. All the physical symptoms of aging are caused by a double-whammy: our hormone levels drop off and our systems can no longer defend against toxins. There is help. The doctor will offer medications with a zillion side effects or you and I can learn about health and practice, safely, on our aging selves.

Two similar affirmations about our health seem positive, but is either really?

"I am healthier than I think I am." True, but this person is apt to worry about every little twinge, ache and new spot on the skin, rather than believe this truth.

Follow Others: Aging Wisdom from Beatitudes, Nature, Kinfolk

"I think I am healthier than I am." Probably false, since this person will ignore every symptom the body presents, and not want to know the truth.

Below are some major conditions that all those aging will recognize to some degree. Included are suggestions where to research simple work-rounds to help maintain good health—actually to forestall the aging process of these five unsightly culprits. Read below and refer to the suggestions for research.

The skin blabs. The skin is our largest organ. Is it any surprise then that it is the first to warn about our health? Aging skin is more than liver spots, wrinkles, sags and folds. These are announcements that the body is no longer filled to the brim with youth. I suspect we all have looked around and jealously noted the smooth, muscular tone of limbs on a young man or woman. This may send us scurrying to the gym for weights or back to sports like basketball. We invest in a fitbit-type tracker or an exercise machine. Nothing wrong with that! But youth is more than skin and muscle. Consider researching: Anti-oxidants; Natural hormones/alternatives.

The neck sags. I had an older teacher in high school who sported a turkey-neck. Shame on me for being repulsed, especially now that my own neck follows suit. For the last two decades, I practiced a stretching-the-neck grimace to help tighten those delicate muscles. It probably held the sags at bay, but time marches on and muscle tone loss indicates that hormones have flown the coop. Consider researching: Stretching vs. Botox; Tightening creams; Collagen.

Follow Others: Aging Wisdom from Beatitudes, Nature, Kinfolk

The hair thins. I met a woman who had a face lift while in her 50s or 60s. I couldn't guess her age until I noticed how short, dry and brittle her hair was. Thin hair dates us, whether dyed or gray. In my 70s, my hair doesn't grow as fast as it used to, and my scalp shows through the hair on the back of my head. Darn hand-held mirrors! Consider researching: Hair vitamins; Saw Palmetto (for women too); Vitamin A & D.

The hips ache. Did we have hip replacement(s) when in our forties and fifties? Why should they begin to cause pain once again in the decades following. Nutrient absorption requires hormones, which are now diminishing. Much can be done to improve our physical environment and to naturally deliver the best nutrition to our bones. Consider researching: Homeopathic remedies; Arnica and T-relief (formerly Traumeel); Orthopedic Issues/Hip Exercises; Orthopedic Buying Tips; Diabetes screening when legs ache; Bursitis and B-12.

Immunity slumps. Oh my, yes! That's why seniors are encouraged to line up at the doctor's office or pharmacy to get their shots against shingles, flu and pneumonia. Nutritional companies tout the advantages of anti-oxidants such as Vitamins E and C. Do they just want your Social Security dollars or is there actual proof that either approach works? Don't forget to check if this immunity change is a side effect of a prescription drug or OTC product you are currently taking. Consider researching: Antioxidants; Blood type; Herbal remedies. See Autoimmune Diseases below.

Autoimmune Diseases. In autoimmune diseases, the body's immune system is turned against various organs of the body. For example, attacking the nervous system (MS) or against the gut (Chrohn's).

Follow Others: Aging Wisdom from Beatitudes, Nature, Kinfolk

Minority groups may experience Rheumatoid Arthritis or Lupus. Hashimoto's disease and Grave's disease are likely causes of thyroid issues. Fibromyalgia is a less-known auto-immune disease that is extremely painful.

Aging may trigger some autoimmune diseases; vice versa, having such a disease may contribute to Diabetes Mellitus.

Tips to try: Be aware of trigger factors; for example, viral infections or sun light (Lupus); Healthy diet; gluten-free; Selenium, 200 mcg capsule daily – my granddaughter's Hashimoto stabilized in two months; Vitamin D3, 10,000iu capsule daily; Natural pain remedies: See pain management in chapter 14.

Memory hides. This sleight-of-hand trick begins around the age of fifty. Well, actually we women are somewhat to blame for its capricious ways. According to C.S. Lewis, women very seldom use a noun. We say enigmatic things like "put that away up there" until our spouses thoroughly dislike to help. We all forget our keys and have to retrace our steps to remember what we search for, but has this gotten worse as the decades roll along? And always the fear of Alzheimer's or dementia lurks in the background. Your odds in this battle with enemies of healthy mental aging can be improved with nutrition. See Other Brain Issues section below.

Age-related Temporary Memory Loss. It is very common for elderly people to begin to forget things. Oh, anyone can get distracted and misplace their keys. The type of memory loss that is related to aging diseases can result in inability to recall words and facts, forgetting days of the week and the monetary value of a quarter, memory of the past but not the present or inability of the brain to communicate commands to the body parts that enable motion.

Follow Others: Aging Wisdom from Beatitudes, Nature, Kinfolk

At the age of fifty, most people begin to experience the temporary inability to recall a certain word/groups, such as nouns. For example, you may try to remember the name of a specific flower, or the name of that person you saw and should know. Never good at people's names, I go easy on myself. Although when not able to remember the name for a flower I used to know, it is frustrating.

According to a Brain Aging video, the healthy brain still stores long-term information. However, as we age the brain's ability to sort quickly for recall doesn't function as well. So instead of just the one wanted name, many other items come up simultaneously, causing the temporary feeling of confusion.

I have learned to expect the missing information to show up sometime within a few days, when I'm least expecting it. Otherwise, I use my cell phone and the internet to hunt it down. Brainstorming with a friend can jog memories, too. Suggesting a synonym verbally is my latest method to trigger a lost noun.

Author C.S. Lewis pointed out that men cannot work well with women because of women's infuriating habit of un-descriptive commands like: "Put this up on the shelf inside of that." Women, we are warned about the habit of not using nouns when we speak. Maybe that's why nouns are the easiest to forget.

Tips to boost memory: B-6; B-12; Exercise by reading complicated materials regularly; Herbs – Gingko (blood type A); Caffeine

For other ways to boost memory, read Dr. Daniel Amen's book on Memory Rescue. His team uses Brain Spect Scans to X-ray for brain trauma or addictions that can harm memory. Consider researching: B vitamins, especially B-6 and B-12; Avoid or limit aluminum contact with food, drinks or skin contact with underarm deodorants; Prevagen and other OTC options.

Follow Others: Aging Wisdom from Beatitudes, Nature, Kinfolk

Alzheimer's /Dementia – Consult a doctor immediately. Some have linked Alzheimer's disease to the use of aluminum pans or wrap, and deodorants. Large parts of the brain have lost brain matter. On the other hand, dementia may be linked to hardening of arteries and even allergic reactions to black mold.

Sufferers may be able to remember names and events from their youth only. My mother-in-law who had Alzheimer's didn't recognize her grown grandchildren who came to visit her. She confused their children with them. A doctor will question the patient and family on details that should be easily remembered. Based on the answers, a probable diagnosis will be made. Autopsy of the deceased's brain provides the only definitive diagnosis for Alzheimer's disease.

Tips that may postpone symptoms: Don't use underarm deodorant with aluminum salts. Natural stone versions safely remove underarm bacteria and eliminate orders (Alzheimer's); Take Vitamins B-6 and B-12 for memory support; Check if anemic; take a multiple with iron and folic acid; Cut out fatty foods (Dementia); Investigate issues with wetness and black mold in the home (Dementia); Keep hydrated (Dementia).

Tips for caregivers: Engage seniors with music, activities requiring short attention span, touch, smells, family recipes; Never argue with, lecture or say "you can't" to patient (Alzheimer's).

Parkinson's Disease – Consult a doctor immediately. Symptoms include small, shuffling steps (B-12); stooped posture, trouble turning around. Doctor will treat with Levodopa (L-dopa) or deep brain stimulation (inactivate parts of brain over stimulated). Note: ordinary shaking as you age is due to stress. Take magnesium and B-6 to reduce stress.

Follow Others: Aging Wisdom from Beatitudes, Nature, Kinfolk

Tips that might prevent Parkinson's: Water exercise, aerobics, laps; Prevent falls – remove loose wires/cords, rugs; Eat healthy – high fiber, whole grains, fresh fruit; Limit fat, sugars, salt; Blood type O more susceptible; blood type A less susceptible.

Major systems go on strike. A dear ninety-three year old man told me that when you hit your eighties, the whole system goes to ****. We can starve these organs literally by feeding them junk. We can traumatize them with alcohol and other addictive substances. We can remain stationary and weaken them with inactivity. We can ignore research to find what works best for us personally—based on our blood type or genetic background. Consider researching: Diets for strongest gland and fat locations indicated by blood types; Eye issues and remedies; Prebiotics. See System Issues—Thyroid and Autoimmune Diseases section below. Kidney and Heart issues may show up, as well; see Chapter 11.

Hypothyroid versus Hyperthyroid. The Thyroid is a small endocrine gland located at the base of the throat. Hypothyroid is a condition where the gland produces too little of the regulating hormone (Hashimoto' disease). Hyperthyroid occurs when the gland produces too much of this hormone (Graves' Disease).

Here are some scenarios that can cause thyroid issues: Cyst or small nodules on the Thyroid or Parathyroid; Result of Hashimoto's disease or Graves' disease (see Autoimmune Diseases above); Too much carbohydrates and sugar, which act like drugs to over-stimulate and tire out this gland. See Dr. Abravanel's Diet plan in chapter 11.

Blood tests can predict the type of thyroid issue; for example, people with Parathyroid issues will test extremely low in Calcium. If surgery is necessary, the person may be prescribed Thyroid hormones for the rest

Follow Others: Aging Wisdom from Beatitudes, Nature, Kinfolk

of their life. Thyroid issues can affect blood pressure readings. See section on Cardio Vascular/Heart Health.

Natural tips to try: Kelp contains Iodine that is needed by the thyroid gland. Kelp is available in tablet format or in packets of seaweed, both available at a health food store; Selenium; CAUTION: add this nutrient prior to kelp, especially for Hashimoto's disease; Avoid stress; If your thyroid is your strongest gland, for breakfast substitute protein, such as eggs, and decaffeinated beverages rather than breads and cereals. Limit yourself to a half slice bread at a sitting. Avoid caffeine unless your adrenal gland is the strongest.

Stroke – Consult a doctor immediately. A blockage to blood flow in the brain is the known cause of strokes. This can result from high blood pressure and stress/overwork. Typically only half of the body is affected due to the location where the brain blockage occurs. Small strokes, called TIAs, may cause the person to temporarily blank out or fall. The person may feel all right afterwards.

Look for lopsided responses; left arm vs. right, one side of the face only. WARNING: If noticed, have the person get to a hospital immediately. If a stroke victim receives treatment within three hours, all effects from the stroke can be reversed. That is why the ability to recognize a stroke is extremely important.

Tests for stroke: Ask the person to smile; Ask the person to talk and also to state a complete sentence; Ask the person to raise both arms; Ask the person to stick out their tongue.

"The idea of living a long life appeals to everyone, but the idea of getting old doesn't appeal to anyone." Andy Rooney

Follow Others: Aging Wisdom from Beatitudes, Nature, Kinfolk

Develop a Counter-Attack Plan

As said earlier, there are three ways to build, or restore, health via: positive thinking; nutrition; exercise. Previous chapters cover positive thinking; this chapter and several that follow will address ways to correct nutritional and exercise deficits/issues.

Whatsoever We Eat – Nutrition

Have you noticed yourself craving things, like sugar, chocolate or salt, that you never liked when young? My mother-in-law in her 60s discovered her diabetes because she began to drink soda by the cans-full for the first time. I could never eat sugar; as a kid I used to hide most of my dessert in the cupboard, but my sister always found and ate it first. With late-onset diabetes a factor in my family, my current toleration of sweets is worrisome.

The food groups we refused to eat as kids, like fruit and vegetables, were needed by the body to flood it with nutrients. Does that mean we can immediately begin to eat all that "good stuff" and turn around the aging process? No, but we probably can find palatable, organic substitutes with better nutrients/content. Most certainly we should learn how to supplement our diets with vitamins, minerals and protein powders. See Vitamin Basics in this chapter.

My background in nutritional healing stems from a fascination with chemistry, physics/ergonomics and a desire from a young age to become a doctor. Leaving college after my freshman year, I never became a chemist as planned, but I still think like one regarding health. I refuse to stop with symptoms and continue to research until learning what is the actual cause of the issue. For example, if your hips hurt is it because the calcium/magnesium ratio is off; or are your b-vitamins out

Follow Others: Aging Wisdom from Beatitudes, Nature, Kinfolk

of balance? Is this a physical condition being aggravated by the poor ergonomics of your computer chair, recliner, or driver's seat? Have your shoe heels run over or do you need arches? I learned from the business world that manufacturers do not design furniture for short people or those with short-waists—all crash dummies are fabricated with long-waists. Everyone has a degree of arthritis, so don't expect that an operation will heal your problems. It may. But why start with a drastic measure when this book has so many other options for you to consider?

One of the most important things I learned is that what works for one person may not work for another. Some people are allergic to prescription medication; you may be, too. Kinesiology can tell if you are. Your family may, like mine, have a high need for vitamin A if the back of your arms in youth were all bumps and pimples. Don't let a professional say it is from taking too frequent baths. We must take the time to get to know our own body.

Isn't There An Easier Way? – Exercise

I am good for short bursts of exercise. I can run, climb steep trails, exercise on my elliptical trainer and swim a few strokes. Just don't expect me to exercise very long. Matter of fact, don't expect me to vacuum the living and dining room rugs without at least two breaks for water, vitamin C (for dust allergies) or snacks. Rearranging furniture becomes a stalling tactic for me.

Recently I have learned about two physical limitations that contribute to this anomaly, one at least I have had my entire life. 1) My adrenal gland is my strongest endocrine gland. That makes short bursts a breeze, but then I tire out quickly. Since I stop an exercise before 20 minutes elapses, it means that my muscles never memorize how to produce over longer periods of time. 2) I recently learned that high blood pressure over the years has caused the apex of my heart to

Follow Others: Aging Wisdom from Beatitudes, Nature, Kinfolk

harden. It can't pump as much blood as normal into the lower ventricles. The doctor says this is not life threatening, but it further limits exercise.

Should I give up? Not a chance. I wanted a Fitbit-type tracker for Christmas and next year plan to climb for a second time to the top of a 800 ft mountain peak on a 1.2 mile trail. Why? In order to hunt for quartz and tourmaline crystals. Seriously? With a walking stick if my hip replacement heals completely by then. (Update: didn't climb another mountain but did purchase a Fitbit-type device.)

Consider researching: Tai Chi and pool exercise – builds core muscles; Silver sneakers programs with most gyms and senior insurance memberships; Family stories, such as Aunt Nina and Prophecy in this chapter.

Must I Smile?

People have told me all my life that I have a nice smile. I didn't figure out until lately that what they politely implied is that when I don't smile, my face looks like the Grinch. My ex-husband taught me the neck exercises I've done for decades; recently my spouse told me to smile more. Think they were pointing something out to me?

Consider researching: Face and neck muscle exercises; Creams that tighten or plump skin that sagged; Collagen. See Youth Restorers in this chapter

Follow Others: Aging Wisdom from Beatitudes, Nature, Kinfolk

Vitamin Basics

How did vitamins get their name? In Europe and America research scientists were learning about how the body is nourished and powered. They discovered elements for life that a Polish biochemist named Casmir Funk called 'vitamines'. In America, Dr. Forrest Shaklee had his Vitalized Minerals at the same time. Shaklee corresponded with the biochemist and both men recognized that nutrition could help prevent deficiency disorders.

Funk is credited with discovery of individual 'vitamines'. Shaklee felt this was an idea whose time had come, to which others—like himself—contributed their knowledge. In 1915 Shaklee first introduced his Vitalized Minerals into his practice.

Synthetic vitamins masquerade. During World War II, synthetic vitamins were manufactured. A synthetic vitamin is the mirror-image of a natural vitamin. Although named almost the same as the natural vitamin, the full name tells the difference. For example, natural vitamin E is known as d-alpha tocopheryl; the synthetic vitamin E is called dl-alpha tocopheryl and it shows up in less expensive vitamin E products. The added L indicates this is a synthetic.

Energy at Expense of Health. To demonstrate why "L" is used in the name of a synthetic vitamin, hold out both of your hands with palms facing you. The right hand illustrates the natural vitamin; the left hand demonstrates the synthetic masquerader. They look nearly identical but the body can recognize the difference. The biggest difference is in how the body responds to the two. The synthetic version triggers an immune response similar to ingestion of any foreign substance. This revs up your body and produces energy. However, the body only is fed and nourished by the natural vitamin.

Follow Others: Aging Wisdom from Beatitudes, Nature, Kinfolk

Multiple vs. Individual Vitamins. When you look at shelf after shelf of vitamins in the drug store, health food store or big box stores, do you ever wonder where to start? I started with individual vitamins, but within a few years learned the importance of a good multiple vitamin.

What's a good multiple supplement? One that is made from the highest quality sources and includes low potency B-vitamins.

Highest quality— means a balance between vitamins and nutrients as well as combinations versus single ingredients. It also means not synthetic (see above) and from non-polluted sources. The company that produces the multiple I take will actually import quality ingredients if local ones are toxic due to exhaust fumes, etc.

Low potency B-vitamins— mean that the body will accept the combination of B's as if from a natural source. High potency B vitamins cause the body to throw out extras, including the very vitamin your body is lowest in. B-12 tablets should be sublingual (dissolve under tongue). Tricky B-vitamins, indeed.

Why take individual vitamins? No matter how balanced a multiple may be, it cannot be customized fully to your individual needs. For example, your family may have a high need for vitamin B-6 or even vitamin A in the winter time. To make a safe multiple, companies follow guidelines suitable for typical needs. Individual vitamins let you troubleshoot by adding more of what your body personally needs. I have a high need for folic acid, a B-vitamin regulated by federal law. Since only 400 mcg is permitted in a multiple, I must purchase this vitamin in larger potencies and take a tablet daily along with my multiple. I also need higher vitamin A in the winter. Individual vitamins allow me to customize.

Follow Others: Aging Wisdom from Beatitudes, Nature, Kinfolk

How to monitor your vitamin intake. (FYI, I presented this method verbally to a pharmacist who agreed with my recommendations.)

Sequence/Analysis:

Take a new vitamin for two weeks. Within that time blame EVERYTHING unusual on the new vitamin—from pimples on the face to constipation. If the consequences are serious, stop the vitamin. If not, continue to take it for two more weeks.

At the end of four weeks, evaluate results. Ask yourself these questions: Do I feel better? Do I feel worse? Is there no noticeable change? Depending on your answers, do one of these:

Stop the vitamin if you feel worse; ask for a refund; Stop the vitamin if you notice no change. Wait two more weeks.

Continue the vitamin if you notice positive results. Wait two more weeks.

At the end of six weeks, ask yourself if things seem better or worse. You may have missed a positive or negative issue that wasn't noticed earlier, such as a few inches lost from your waist. Make the decision to include, restore or discontinue the new vitamin/supplement.

As I write this book, I am amazed when comparing my Resources list with the most current information found online. Things I was guided to study about in the 1970s are as valid now as at the beginning of America's search for nutritional health. I was tickled to see on Amazon the covers of nearly-ancient cookbooks I once knew well and used to collect many favorite recipes.

Why should anyone care about "ancient" health history? Knowing this information provides us the basis to evaluate current fads and facts and to keep our health on a steady keel. Without basic facts, we must

Follow Others: Aging Wisdom from Beatitudes, Nature, Kinfolk

continually make subjective decisions that may lead us to waffle, weave and possibly take an online tangent that can seriously impact our chances of healthy aging.

I was interested in nutrition before it became fashionable. I know why something works, how to decide what is best and what is bogus. Now in my late-seventies I wish to pass this information along as my legacy to others.

Youth Restorers. Have you ever observed a child and wondered where all the energy comes from? Or can you remember late nights out and still ready for a full-day's work in the morning? How does youth manage? The answer is simple; their bodies still manufacture key nutrients that keep them young and active.

Both COQ10 and L-Carnitine are popular nowadays. The bodies of seniors still produce small amounts of each of these substances. However, aging people have decreased levels. That's why supplementation from the age of forty-plus can improve energy levels and heart health.

WARNING: If you are under doctor's care for any condition, discuss the content of this document with your professional. Medications may need to be adjusted as your health improves.

CoQ10 in pill or liquid format. This nutrient is produced in our bodies and has antioxidant properties which protect cells from damage by free radicals that accompany the aging process. Free radicals notably attack skin, heart and brain cells.

My experience: My heart doctor in the 1980s told me to read the book "Heart Sense for Women" and take both of these youth restorers. I struggled with high blood pressure, made worse by white coat

Follow Others: Aging Wisdom from Beatitudes, Nature, Kinfolk

syndrome (visits at doctor's office). Once I added the Ubiquinol version of COQ10, I noticed an increase in my energy level; I wasn't tired out after 40-hour work weeks.

L-Carnitine. This amino acid helps build body protein. Good for heart health as well as muscle issues.

My experience: I can't remember why I didn't start the recommended L-Carnitine at the same time. I do remember when and why I finally did start. I was out of work after the dot.com bust, and was busy with some renovations in our two-story country farmhouse. One day around 2004 I felt out of breath as I washed dishes. I noticed the same feeling on a walk when my arms swung at my side. I pulled out the "Heart Sense for Women" book and began to search for what it said about this condition. Aha, Dr. Sinatra recommended L-Carnitine. I bought some and added it to my vitamin regime immediately. The next week I could scour wallpaper from a bedroom wall. No issues with breathing; I was convinced!

Aunt Nina and Prophecy

She was nearly blind when I first met this great aunt. Older than her husband, Edwin Corliss, Nina could only read if the paper was within an inch of her eyes, but that never stopped her. She travelled with my great uncle to Massachusetts where she researched town hall records to find details of his Corliss genealogy—long before online genealogies were available. Then Aunt Nina published it in hardcover in 1964. All her research was done prior to Ancestry.com.

These were the loves of Aunt Nina's life:

She loved the Corliss name, the first ancestor arrived from England in 1635, five years before Ralph Waldo Emerson's forebear. Both of these

Follow Others: Aging Wisdom from Beatitudes, Nature, Kinfolk

noteworthy Puritan families lived north of Boston until my Corliss relatives moved to Vermont in the 1800s. Emerson and Corliss relatives fought in the American revolution. So, I qualify as a documented member of the Daughters of the American Revolution (DAR).

She loved birds—from canaries to parakeets. They shared her living room in elegant cages. Their warble or songs were so lovely it almost made me wish I had the 'pet gene'. The death of one of those birds warned my mother while in her teens of a gas leak and saved her life. After I noticed that paper lined the bottom of the cage and had to be removed regularly, my attitude toward owning a bird changed. I'm such a wimp that I bought a Victorian cage, but keep it purely for decoration.

Aunt Nina loved Biblical prophecy, especially the Old Testament book of Daniel, more than anyone I ever met. She expected within 40 years (one generation) of Israel's birth as a state that the end time prophecies would be fulfilled. She loaned me a book to read about the names assigned to the stars of the Zodiac. I was amazed to see how these ancient names predicted that a savior born of a virgin would become king.

Aunt Nina lived until 90; she did instill within me her interest in prophecy, though not pets. I never was as devoted as she to Bible prophecy, but the last forty years I have watched the newspapers/reports with keen interest. Might this or that world event hold any prophetic consequence? The book of Revelations states that the whole world will watch, at the same moment, a future event in Jerusalem. This was not possible until the satellite communication systems those and other brave men pioneered.

Follow Others: Aging Wisdom from Beatitudes, Nature, Kinfolk

When I wrote my book, "Miracle of the Call" stories of seventeen heroes of the twentieth century, I pointed out that the Wright Brothers and Neil Armstrong both grew up in Dayton, and their aeronautical feats happened less than seventy years apart. The moon landing, celebrating its 50th anniversary in 2019, was the first event all peoples of the world could watch at the same time.

End Point: Follow the recommended research points given throughout this chapter.

Prayer Point: Beatitude according to Luke—Blessed are ye that weep now: for ye shall laugh. Luke 6:21b

Follow Others: Aging Wisdom from Beatitudes, Nature, Kinfolk

Beatitude: Blessed—happy, enviably fortunate, and spiritually prosperous [that is, possessing the happiness produced by experience of God's favor and especially conditioned by the revelation of his grace, regardless of their outward conditions]—are the pure in heart, for they shall see God! Matthew 5:8 Amplified

Chapter 7—External Aging is Universal

"But they that wait upon the LORD shall renew their strength; they shall mount up with wings as eagles; they shall run, and not be weary; and they shall walk, and not faint." Isaiah 40:31

My mother always had thin, straight hair. Fortunately, permanent waves were in fashion then. When she grew older, I remember her additional complaints about thinning hair. Like the irritating know-it-all I could be, I simply advised, against her church, to cut it short. She would have the last laugh now, as my once full-head of hair has thinned down, too. Oh, I still have some bouncy waves she never had, but nowadays my ponytail resembles a pig's tail.

Some of us will begin to age earlier than others, likely due to genetics. Except for accidental death (or the rapture), we will all experience at least a few of the health issues mentioned in the next sections. At the end of this section there is a list of targeted natural remedies that may work for you. For specific aging issues for males and females, see the next chapter.

This chapter and the next offer some natural tips worth considering; they may provide a measure of health as you age.

"Jesus went about..healing all kinds of sickness and all kinds of disease among the people." Matthew 4:23

Follow Others: Aging Wisdom from Beatitudes, Nature, Kinfolk

Caution: For those looking for healing advice, please read the Guidelines and Warning section below. I have not meant this detailed information to supersede advice from a medical professional. The tips offered are generic and cannot possibly take into account your personal health information. However, they will provide you with key words to research online and discuss with your doctor.

Guidelines for Taking Natural Remedies

WARNING: If you try any remedy listed, be aware that delays to see a doctor could hinder diagnosis and timely intervention for serious issues! If you are under doctor's care for any condition, discuss the content of this document with that professional. Medications may need to be adjusted as your health improves.

IMPORTANT: It is always best to consult with a doctor or medical professional to get a proper diagnosis. If the medicine prescribed does not work for you, that is the point when it is alright to try one of the natural remedies mentioned in this chapter, as per the recommendations below (in fact, this is similar to appropriate procedure to try a new pharmaceutical medication):

Take the prescribed dosage per the bottle. If it makes you feel ill, stop immediately. Otherwise, try for two weeks. If the issue has gotten worse, stop at the 2-week mark. Blame everything from pimples to constipation on the remedy. If your issue is improved or at least not gotten worse, continue for two more weeks.

If there is no improvement at one month, stop the remedy. Go to next step. If nothing worse, continue to take for two more weeks.

At six weeks, add this to your regular regimen if improvement is noticed. Or if results are not obvious, stop the remedy and re-evaluate in a month; you may have missed a change.

Follow Others: Aging Wisdom from Beatitudes, Nature, Kinfolk

Ask yourself these questions: Do I have more or less pain? Am I better able to stick to a diet and eat well? Have I lost inches off my waist if not weight? Did some issue go away? Has a new issue developed?

IMPORTANT. Does any prescription medication need adjusting? If yes, see your doctor as soon as possible.

Exterior Aging – Generic

"Remember..the Creator in the days of..youth while the evil days draw not close..when keepers tremble, strong men bow themselves, grinders cease, windows be darkened..because man goes to his long home." {paraphrase of Ecclesiastes 12: 1-7]

Hair and Nail To-dos

"Both the gray-haired and very aged are among us..much older than your father." Job 15:10

Salt and pepper hair is 50% gray; pure white is 100% gray. The front half of my hair is near 100% while the back of my head is somewhere near 80%, I'd guess. As we age it is vital to take good care of our hair. And haircuts above the shoulder line look best.

Four Hair Types. Years ago I read a book by Oprah's hair dresser on hair types. He mentioned four hair types, with recommended styles and techniques for each. I recently researched the section on gray hair. These hair types are updated below for senior hair.

Straight – gray hair has more body; Care: wash daily, use blue shampoo occasionally, clear or blue gels only to style; geometric cuts recommended.

Follow Others: Aging Wisdom from Beatitudes, Nature, Kinfolk

Wavy – type where hair ends always resemble the letter "S". Ends turn upward until long enough to turn under and repeat. Make sure cut length doesn't accentuate saggy neck; Care: wash and condition every other day; wet in between; blunt cut with or w/o highlights, or one long layer near shoulder line.

Curly – resembles a slinky with curls along the length of the hair shaft; curl pattern changes with gray, high humidity will frizz; Care: wet hair every day, shampoo every other day, alcohol-free mousse or gel; cut above shoulder line.

Kinky – tightly-curled, very fragile, can wear hair long; Care: wash once or twice a week with protein-based shampoo, condition every time; avoid repeated heat; natural short curl or straightened bob.

Thinning Hair. I wore my long hair up in a bun for seventeen years. The thin area just above my forehead reminds me that hair pulled too tight when young can have later consequences.

Here are some other suggestions (beside my mother's permanent wave): Pick and choose a shampoo that claims to nourish hair for fuller body; Apply conditioner only to hair ends to avoid weighting down the top; If possible, part hair to cover any bald areas; Wear a hat that doesn't flatten your hair, but any hat is better than catching cold, getting pneumonia, sun stroke or face cancer. I'm an extremist, remember?

Chin Hair/Mustache/Legs. One place where there is more hair after aging begins is facial hair for women. We can all call to mind a comic picture of this on the internet. Men don't fare much better since their facial hair usually turns traitorously white soon after the temples do. Women's legs and underarms do sport less body hair.

Follow Others: Aging Wisdom from Beatitudes, Nature, Kinfolk

Options for women: Clip to remove chin and moustache hair growth; Wax or have unsightly hair permanently removed; Less need to shave legs

Options for men: Keep chin hair closely cropped; Wear chin hair long and braided—no matter the color (ala "redneck" or motorcycle rider); dye/color facial hair until totally gray.

Turning Gray. Anyone who shops during the weekday, morning to mid-afternoon, will notice that a majority of the people have gray/white hair. That's because we retirees, both men and women, are out in force—no longer ashamed to a sport full gray hair-do.

Although it may be hard to remember your original hair color, this will determine your gray hair color:

No red=silver/gray

Redhead=blonde; my mother-in-law was a redhead and blonde in the same lifetime!

Brunette with red=platinum blonde

Coloring Hair. Raise your hand if you ever colored your dark hair to cover gray. Most hands go up, even the men. Nowadays, hair color change is fashionable for the young and considered necessary for professionals competing with younger generations in the work place.

For the aging, most of us breathe a sigh of relieve when we no longer have to color. That relief lasts for awhile if you are lucky enough to have one of the lovely shades of gray (see above). Since my hair was never a single color, all white hair does not interest me in the least. I effuse over the vibrant blues and pinks of the brave, young shop clerks

Follow Others: Aging Wisdom from Beatitudes, Nature, Kinfolk

who wait on me. The question remains: will I get brave enough to try color again.

Low Lights vs. High Lights. I have it straight from the hairdresser's mouth that I cannot add highlights to my hair. White hair is a highlight. Instead, I can add low lights, darker tones streaked in to add dimension to a gray head. I hoped this could be a temporary scenario, in case I hate the outcome. Since low lights have to be permanent hair coloring, I might get adventurous some winter when I get my customary blunt cut to clear the tops of my turtle necks. Check back in the Spring!

Fingernails/Toenails. Nails are made of keratin, a hard protein that is also found in hair. Our nails are indicators of overall health. As we age we will notice some changes in the nails including:

Ridges – Horizontal (can indicate health problems) or vertical (normal sign of aging)

White flecks in the nail bed (low in zinc)

Brittle nails

Yellow color (can indicate fungus or trauma)

Separation of nail from nail bed

Infection around cuticles

IMPORTANT: Arrange a physical with your doctor if any of these nail changes are noted. Diabetes can often produce nail problems. MRSA can cause cuticle infections that require an antibiotic. Check large black streak under toenail immediately; it could be cancerous.

Follow Others: Aging Wisdom from Beatitudes, Nature, Kinfolk

Aging Skin: Early Signs

"You have filled me with wrinkles..my leanness has risen up and bears witness to my face." Job 16:8

Skin Undertones. Coloring, and no I don't mean black versus white, but rather pink, yellow or sallow undertones which we all have. The 1980s saw the popularity of the "Color Me Beautiful" book, swatches and theory of Carole Jackson. You could guess yourself or go for a color consultation to learn whether you were a Winter, Spring, Summer or Fall. This is determined by your unique combination of skin tones, eye color and hair color. Of course, we could be possessors of mismatched red hair and blue eyes (Summer) instead of brown (Autumn). Recently, I spoke to someone about how to choose colors. Like a true Winter person, she stuck to neutrals with only a pop of color. Carole Jackson explained in the 1980s that we all can wear color, but it must be the right shade of blue, pink or yellow, etc.

Best Aging Color Choices. Why bring up this outdated strategy for choice of clothing colors? For two reasons related to aging.

Reason number one: Sallow skin. Your skin color changes when you age. And the new color of those in the 70s or greater is a yellow-gray commonly known as sallow. One remedy for this condition is to use a colored moisturizer or makeup with more pink than you used to wear. It does make a difference. I will never have a photo taken again without a pink highlighter applied first! Read Color Me Sallow section below.

Reason number two: Right Shade. How do you recognize the right shade for aging skin? Hold a garment up to your face and look in the mirror. If your eyes look at the garment, it's wrong for you. If your eyes look at your face it is the right color for you. But there's more.

Follow Others: Aging Wisdom from Beatitudes, Nature, Kinfolk

Choosing the right color can surprisingly bring in the aging factor. If I wear black near my face, because it goes perfectly with my Winter coloring, it draws eyes to my wrinkles. Do I really want that? Maybe pick charcoal gray instead of black or less dynamic shades of favorite colors that will not cause such contrast.

Choosing the wrong color is easier to fix. With my brown eyes, I like some Autumn colors. If I hold up a rust colored (Autumn) dress when in front of a mirror, I quickly notice that it makes my face look older than if I hold up a magenta (Winter) blouse. Watch for that aging factor when buying clothes.

You know what? It might not be a bad idea to pull that dusty copy of "Color Me Beautiful" down from the book shelf for another go around. Or check the author's web site: http://carolejacksoncolors.com/

Color Me Sallow. What is sallow skin and is it a sign of aging? I noticed one winter that the skin of my face looked dingy. I learned this was because the pink glow had left with age and the yellow undertones were showing. Apparently, this was also a sign that my body wasn't healthy—not necessarily a sign of aging. The fact was that one of my blood pressure medications caused pneumonia like symptoms that left a cough for months. I even cracked a rib with the coughing.

So what can we do to return the rosy pink tones once they fade? First of all, my Mom was English (rose tones) and my Dad was Italian (yellow tones). These tones neutralized each other and I always had beige skin except when tanned at summertime. Nowadays the yellow wins.

I found on the internet several things I can do to right my skin tone:

Use creamy cleanser, anti-oxidant serums, SPF Moisturizer and clay mask weekly. Twice a day cleanse/moisturize routines are mandatory. How does our body always know when we skimp?

Follow Others: Aging Wisdom from Beatitudes, Nature, Kinfolk

Drink enough water to stay hydrated inside; important for wrinkles, too. Ditto on the skimp.

Quit smoking - You should anyways; thankfully I never did.

Get the recommended hours of sleep.

Take a high-quality, low-potency B-vitamin complex to stay stress free. B vitamins need to be taken together in proper balance.

Make sure to get enough iron-rich foods.

If all else fails, you can do what I did. Buy a pink, color-correct primer and apply it over your moisturizer. I never forget to do that when I will be photographed.

Feed the Skin. Skin is the largest organ of your body and has definite preferences about what you should feed it. Since King Solomon's reign, as well as Cleopatra's, there have been formulations applied to the body before or after a bath. Romans were known for their baths; they built bath houses in every city they conquered. Books are available that give recipes to prepare your own home skin care treatments. And there are stores in the largest malls and online that cater to the rich and the stars.

Recommended strategies to feed your skin:

Apply the most natural skin creams you can afford.

Choose cosmetics that are right for your skin type, not necessarily your age. Your skin may be much younger than you are chronologically, or older if you neglected it.

If you cannot tolerate fragrances or harsh cleansers, look for labels that say "Hypoallergenic".

Follow Others: Aging Wisdom from Beatitudes, Nature, Kinfolk

Use natural lint-free wipes or face clothes to apply or remove creams from your skin.

Apply an SPF factor moisturizer on hands and face daily.

Vary the skin creams you use regularly. I use two kinds alternated several times a week. I don't like to eat the same foods regularly. Why would my skin, and largest organ, not appreciate a palate change?

Warnings: Avoid applying skin creams to broken skin; Toss out cosmetics with applicators, or samples, within two years or less.

Aging Skin Structure. Skin cells regenerate about every five weeks. Damage caused by poor nutrition and sun exposure may improve when corrective measures are taken. However, the aging skin will continue to be more susceptible based on the less-youthful structure explained below.

Thin Skin. What's underneath the skin may intrigue a skin doctor, but the rest of us really don't want to gaze at it often. Unfortunately, aging causes skin to thin. Now every vein shows. Aging spots appear from sun toasted sugars under the skin. And small blood vessels (purpura) rupture in the ankle area. These purpura look like a surface rash, but are visible through the thin skin around ankle bones. These alarmed my daughter (in her thirties then), who asked in worried tones what was wrong with me. Alas younger women, they will show up in your future, too.

Elastin. This highly-elastic protein in connective tissue allows many tissues in the body to resume their shape after being stretched. Guess what happens when age reduces their ability to bounce back? Yup, wrinkles and unsightly skin folds on face and arms. What you can do:

Purchase and use one of the many face creams that claim to restore elastin.

Follow Others: Aging Wisdom from Beatitudes, Nature, Kinfolk

Do facial exercises, including massage and smiling.

Increase intake of protein drinks/powders.

Circle flabby arms while outstretched at side of body.

Find a brand of clothing that sells fashionable three-quarter length sleeves.

Collagen Support. Collagen is the next great thing since sliced bread. And you know what, this may indeed be the missing link to plumper skin on the face and neck. Stop at any health food store and ask questions. Or order online at Amazon. Taken in a drink, hot or cold, once daily can do wonders. I've recently emptied a canister of collagen with noticeable improvement in my unsightly turkey neck and jowls. And I bought a tasteless collagen for the male in my life that dissolves in his hot coffee.

CAUTION: Be sure to read labels before purchase. One brand of collagen powder includes a large amount of coconut products. I suspected that a rash on my throat indicated I might be allergic to frequent coconut intake; I switched to a different brand. However, the real culprit turned out to be shellfish (krill) oil, now being used instead of fish oil in a supplement I had taken for years.

Facial Muscles Tense. Wrinkle patterns on the face indicate health issues. They also indicate facial tension. I'm not much of a 'smiler'. Anyone can read my thoughts on my face. Good nutrition helped prevent wrinkles for awhile, but eventually more is needed.

People tell me I look nicer when I smile. So I've been doing more of that lately. One time in my life, I used to look in my car's side mirror and watch myself smile. Not wise if driving, but I know who to blame

Follow Others: Aging Wisdom from Beatitudes, Nature, Kinfolk

for my love of mirrors. My mother could stop my crying when a young child by giving me a mirror to see how ugly it made me look. Thanks, Mom.

Sun Damage and Dark Spots. The dark spots on hands and face that are often called Liver Spots are really sun damage. Heat causes carbohydrates, sugar and collagen protein under the skin to toast (called glycation). The browned result is one of the compounds called AGEs and is similar to browned edges of meat in a pan.

Cosmetologists claim there are remedies that can be applied twice daily to the skin to remove these dark spots. I tried one, but could not tolerate the product's fragrance. I gave it to a friend to try out. See section on fragrance allergies.

Rosacea. This chronic condition affects people between the ages of 30 and 50. Damage caused by this skin ailment can leave red, scaly patches visible on your pale aging face. I have a small patch where a skin cancer was removed.

Skin Cancer and Vitamin B-6. In my sixties I had a bout of skin cancer incidents. Talk about scary! My skin doctor and I started seeing a lot of each other. Research brought me to a well-read but obscure health book, "Healing Yourself" which I owned since the 1970s. It claimed a lack of B-6 could cause cancer. I took a 100 mg B-6 tablet every day, along with my high-quality, low-potency B-vitamin complex. I've not had another skin cancer since. Stress can affect our Bs and do ugly things with our skin.

IMPORTANT: B vitamins are water soluble and wash out of your system quickly. You need not fear that a single dose of B-6 could cause serious issues. Read section on oily vs. water soluble vitamins.

Follow Others: Aging Wisdom from Beatitudes, Nature, Kinfolk

Skin Tags, Warts, AKs and Miscellaneous Thingies. Aging skin appears to be the ideal home for a variety of non-cancerous lesions and protrusions. Rough or smooth, raised or stuck out like a sore thumb, these seem to show up were clothing aggravates the skin. These protruding thingies may annoy (like your tongue finding a chipped tooth). However, lesions underneath the skin can actually be more serious.

Skin tags are frequent around the collar/neck area or under arm pits. Multiple tags may be associated with diabetes.

Actinic Keratosis (AK) is a precursor to cancer caused by exposure to the sun. I've had these scaly spots irritate and itch areas where bra straps, fasteners and underwire rub. Also, on my abdomen and back.

Warts on the hands or feet are typical; less typical are those that have shown up on my shoulders underneath the bra straps.

Cherry Angiomas are raised up red blood growths most often appearing on the abdomen of women. They result from hormonal changes such as pregnancy and aging and are harmless.

Moles vs. Melanomas

See a skin doctor if you notice any change in color, size or shape of a dark, mole like growth.

An existing mole can become cancerous due to sun exposure. I had a mole from birth on the top of my foot. When I was in my forties, it became a basal cell cancer and had to be removed.

Melanomas are beneath the surface, blue or black in color and not symmetrical. See a skin doctor immediately as these can be life-threatening.

Visits to the Dermatologist. Medicare will pay for health-related visits to a dermatologist. You will be charged only a co-pay if the issue is indeed health-related but not malignant. If malignancy is suspected, the whole charge will be covered. Any cosmetic procedure costs twice that.

Biopsies are done with a knife. Otherwise, the doctor uses a gun to freeze the surface, followed in certain cases by cauterization. These in-office procedures take 2-3 weeks to heal.

Cosmetic Surgery. Perhaps you have already investigated cosmetic surgery around the eyes or a face lift. The costs are not covered by insurance and can be quite expensive. The procedures are susceptible to many of the side effects following any surgery: swelling, redness, infection, bleeding. Hopefully, the results would be worth the effort and expense. I met a woman who claimed she was in her eighties. The face lift she had done was so excellent she looked to be in her fifties. However, her dry, unhealthy hair was that of an eighty-year-old.

Lumps and Bulges

Cysts and Fatty Tumors. Many people have cysts and tumors that grow on their body. Women can have cystic breasts and ovaries. Both sexes have fatty tumors often on the chest—back or front. Not much can be done to remove these lumps. A calcified fatty tumor may impinge on a nerve and have to be removed by minor surgery.

Other people have ganglion cyst(s) that grow on the wrist or parts of the hand. Old medical books say to smash the cyst with a heavy book. I suggest you take the homeopathic remedy; Causticum, a single dose of 30c may have surprising success.

Follow Others: Aging Wisdom from Beatitudes, Nature, Kinfolk

Hernias. Most babies are born with a hernia below their umbilical cord. This tear usually causes no trouble until you wear pants too tight around the waist. Adult hernias can result from straining while lifting heavy objects. A tear can allow the intestine to poke through causing external discomfort. Surgery can repair the tear.

Varicose Veins. Any varicose veins you may have in your legs are more visible with aging thin skin.

Wear support hose/stockings

After standing on your feet or shopping, lay in bed with feet toward the headboard. Raise your legs and brace your feet against the wall. This helps the blood to flow upstream back to the heart.

Take vitamin E for increased circulation. Consult with your doctor if already on a blood thinner.

"He has..gathered fat upon his waist." Job 15:27

Abdominal Fat. And note that verse does not have a good connotation. We definitely aren't advised to get fat around the mid-section, and for several good reasons. This is referred to as the apple body shape. Maybe you don't eat many fatty things, but sugars will convert to body fat as well. Here's a list of why we should watch what we eat:

Abdominal fat can aggravate or cause heart conditions.

Too much fat in a diet can cause gall-bladder disease and gall-stones. If your gall-bladder has already been removed, the fat accumulates in your liver. Not good since the liver is our first line of defense against toxins.

Check out fat-burning diet plans in chapter 11.

Follow Others: Aging Wisdom from Beatitudes, Nature, Kinfolk

What you think is fat in the abdomen may be ascites, abnormal buildup of fluid, as a manifestation of ovarian cancer. Check with a doctor, especially if you have lost the desire to eat.

Eye Concerns. Younger folk tend to have near-sighted vision, meaning they can see things better that are up close. I know I was near-sighted, that and a bit of astigmatism (crossed eyes) got me a pair of glasses before high school. My mom wore glasses early, too.

Aging eyes tend to shift to far-sighted vision, which means that they see things farther away best. And there is a rather comical point midway in life when our arms become too short to see well. We're headed toward far-sighted but not off-in-a-distance far sighted yet.

I still need correction for astigmatism and now cataracts, too. But with corrective lenses I can almost see each individual leaf on trees at the horizon. That's far-sighted indeed. Cataracts that are ready for surgery revert your eyes to being nearsighted. I recently dug out an older pair of glasses; the lenses seem to work for now. However, surgery is clearly in my future.

Note to Seniors: at some age your state may insist that you pass an eye exam in order to get your driver's license renewed. Check with your state DMV to ask about this.

Lasik Surgery. Are you a good candidate for corrective Lasik surgery? This procedure can eliminate the need for corrective lenses. However, not everyone will have excellent results. For example, people with large pupils may experience a glow around lit objects, similar to cataracts, after Lasik surgery. Consult with an Ophthalmologist about your options.

Follow Others: Aging Wisdom from Beatitudes, Nature, Kinfolk

Floaters/Detached Retina. Aging people are apt to experience both, one more serious than the other. For me, a new floater appeared after my helmet bounced off the ground when the motorcycle I was riding fell. What caused the previous floaters I cannot say. The detached retina I experienced was due to a spike in blood pressure and stress; this tear healed itself.

Floaters are strings of protein come loose from the gel-like vitreous at the back of the eye. These move around like shadows. When first discovered they may even block the field of view; later they may reposition themselves, or we learn to ignore them.

WARNING: Detached Retina can be a medical emergency. Contact an eye professional as soon as possible.

Retinal detachment is apt to occur after 40. This eye condition occurs when a portion of the light sensitive layer that lines the back of the eye pulls or tears away. There are three levels of detachment, based on the damage done. Some, like me, may see white lines around the edge of the eye; others may experience a black area.

Dry Eyes, Drippy Eyes. Older eyes have irritation issues. My eye lids feel itchy most of the time, especially early morning. Most annoying is the dripping when out in the cold and wind. I was hiking down a hill recently and had to keep my eyes down to avoid tripping over roots in the trail. My eyes dripped into the glass lens and formed puddles there.

Doctors say both these annoyances are caused by dry eyes and is called dry eye syndrome. Nasal sprays and antihistamines can cause drippy eyes. Check the side effects of all medications and OTC remedies you take.

Omega-3 fatty acids should show improvement in three months

Take blink breaks from your monitor

Follow Others: Aging Wisdom from Beatitudes, Nature, Kinfolk

Check side effects of your antihistamine tablet or nasal spray

Dr. Sam Berne recommends eye exercises: Focus off at a distance for a few seconds; then focus at a closer distance. He has a series of online courses on eye care. https://www.drsamberne.com/eye-exercises/

Eye Diseases. There are a whole slew of age-related eye diseases. The most common are discussed in this section. As usual our emphasis is on how to treat aging issues naturally. Tests commonly used to evaluate eye health are pupil-dilation eye drops and puffs of air directed at the eyeball.

IMPORTANT: Always consult with a doctor, optometrist or ophthalmologist to get evaluated before trying natural remedies.

Medical insurance will cover yearly or more frequent consultation with an Ophthalmologist for any of the eye diseases listed below. The insurance will also cover surgery and first pair of eyeglasses post-operative. Do not skimp on such an important issue as your eyesight.

Cataracts – Consult a doctor immediately. A clear lens refracts a single image. In the case of cataracts, the lens becomes opaque, cloudy and develops refractive defects that produce multiple, splintered, starburst or blurry images. Cataracts develop as part of the aging process. However, steroids can cause cataracts to present at an earlier age.

My cataract story started when I had back surgery. After surgery, I tried what was unofficially touted as a "natural pain relief" product. It worked and I took it faithfully for two years. What I didn't realize was that it contained a bovine steroid, and that steroids can cause early-onset cataracts.

I began with seeing a glow around objects. The initial damage to my lenses was apparently too small to be seen, but after a few office visits at my insistence, someone diagnosed cataracts. By that time, headlamps

Follow Others: Aging Wisdom from Beatitudes, Nature, Kinfolk

of cars, as well as light sparkles off of metallic objects, splintered into what I called firecrackers. When my eyes tired, I could see the characteristic halo around these lights.

Now the doctor says I have old-age cataracts. At the moment, they are bad enough to prevent me from driving at night. I can see until an oncoming car shines its lights at me. If a person crossed the street behind that vehicle, I would never see them. Lighted four-lane highways are safer to navigate. Gray on gray or white on black make things indiscernible.

I suspect my current intake of supplements, similar to those found in those recommended for macular degeneration, keep my cataracts from further "ripening." Update: My cataracts are finally ready for surgery, but I'm hoping to put that off until this summer. I've had too many surgeries in the past year to want to sign up right now for another set.

Eye Drops Warning. I heard about MSM and Cineraria eye drops that could help cataracts. I ordered them from Amazon, and only realized when they arrived that they were bottled overseas. I wasn't brave enough to be a guinea pig and test those eye drops in my eyes.

Glaucoma – Consult a doctor immediately. This disease manifests itself as high pressure within the eye ball (intraocular pressure) that can cause damage to the optical nerves of the eye This pressure can be caused if there is blockage that prevents draining of eye fluids per design. This can lead to loss of peripheral vision. Ophthalmologists will prescribe eye drops for the eye(s) to increase outflow of fluid from the eye. Stress can cause Glaucoma.

Macular Degeneration – Consult a doctor immediately. When your mom told you to eat your carrots for your eyes, she spoke the truth. Carotenoids are fat-soluble anti-oxidants that promote eye health. Macular Degeneration is an age-related disease that causes a gray area to appear in the middle of the individual's eye sight. Injections by needle in the eye is the current treatment. Instead:

Follow Others: Aging Wisdom from Beatitudes, Nature, Kinfolk

Take a vitamin supplement especially for eye health. This should include carotenoids, especially lutein (40 mg) and zeaxanthin; Shaklee sells the Carotomax® product to prevent eye problems.

NOTE: Make sure you're not allergic to herbs used in supplements and remedies.

Hearing Loss. Have you reached sixty-five without receiving an invitation/postcard to have your hearing checked? Hearing specialists will still contact you even if you move to another state. They know there's little chance that you won't experience some hearing loss due to aging.

Men seem to have trouble hearing higher-pitched sounds, at least that's what I assume from the fact that they can ignore my soprano tones calling them for dinner. And I think this is a scientific fact. Similarly, women have problems hearing some of the lower tones if there is other noise. I guess that married partners can expect to argue about not being heard/listened to indefinitely—with scientific impunity.

Pay the Penalty for Blasted Music. Young males are notorious for addiction to their loud speakers and music. My sons and their father all wore headphones with music blasting while washing dishes. I was grateful for the help, but unaware of consequences to their hearing later in life.

Fragrance Allergies. Some people like those in my family are intolerant of herbal preparations with fragrance often used in shampoos, conditioners and soaps. We also do not tolerate many fragrances associated with essential oils. I learned some time ago that the dislike of fragrance shows the presence of hives on the brain, which is actually

Follow Others: Aging Wisdom from Beatitudes, Nature, Kinfolk

inflammation of the brain. This could have resulted from medication taken as a child, antibiotics or anesthesia.

If you fit into this category, use extreme care when sampling items with fragrance. Side effects may be difficult to deal with.

Dental Woes. Most have acquired an assortment of dental appliances over a lifetime. I was thankful to have only several crowns and a bridge, but have increased those numbers recently. BTW, I learned that people with blood type A have fewer dental problems than those with other blood types. At least one health advantage in our favor!

Accidents, often from youth, account for some dental issues. I broke a tooth at five years when I fell off the edge of a sandbox; yep, clumsy from way back. I know someone who had two teeth in the front knocked out by a playmate. And someone else got kicked in the face by a dog, but only got a broken nose—no teeth lost. Motto: stay out of the sand box and away from unsocial dogs.

Other dental misfortunes can be teeth loss due to cavities and/or impacted molars. I had a dentist tell me once that my insurance would pay for me to have my jaw broken due to misalignment. Didn't opt for that procedure; I couldn't imagine how to reply to people who asked what was different with my face. I have a bit of TMJ (see below) now since I did not follow the dentist's advice.

Follow Others: Aging Wisdom from Beatitudes, Nature, Kinfolk

Fear of the Dentist. Do you approach a dental visit with fear and trepidation? Of course, most of our fears never materialize. Here are a few facts that might help easy them:

You could be allergic to the pretopical numbing substance, benzocaine, dentists dab on your gum prior to inserting the needle containing Novocain. I am allergic, and benzocaine makes me feel like I will pass out. I always thought I was just anxious. Not so—pure allergic reaction. It's in my dental records now—NO pre-topical.

If you have a bottom tooth pulled, and suck your mouth during the night this may keep the site from healing. Remove the tag from a slightly wet tea bag and gently push it into the hole overnight. You will heal quickly from the tannic acid found in tea. Decaf tea is better if you want to sleep.

If you have dental surgery and suffer with pain for longer than usual and/or have a bad taste, you may have an infection in the bone. Contact your dentist ASAP for a different antibiotic.

Diet Suggestions for Dental Health. Here is a list of do's and don'ts:

Reduce how many sweets you eat. I disliked sugary treats until recently.

Brush twice a day; floss once daily; change tooth brush regularly.

Take folic acid to reduce gum disease; this important B-vitamin is found in green leafy vegetables

Do not use charcoal toothpaste as it might scratch the enamel on your teeth.

Read the section on how to balance Calcium and Magnesium.

Follow Others: Aging Wisdom from Beatitudes, Nature, Kinfolk

Costs and Dental Insurance. What is not funny is the $1000 charge for a crown. This appliance need results from teeth with old fillings that can no longer be replaced due to hairline cracks from chewing. Dental insurance is now a necessity for those who want to Age excellently.

Temporomandibular Joint (TMJ) Disorder. TMJ is no joke. It can be downright painful, and not easily explained why it occurs. Many cases show up or recur after a visit to the dentist, caused from extending the jaw too long or too wide while tense.

My own TMJ incident was caused several years ago at a restaurant. I was a bit disgruntled (more than a bit maybe) as I ate and talked with friends. I opened my mouth wide and heard my jaw crack. The next day it cracked again less loudly, but a nagging point in my temple has taken years to clear. Stress makes this worse. Thankfully it was a minor case.

Dos and Don'ts of TMJ:

See a doctor if jaw pain persists. Or take homeopathic T-Relief.

Do gentle exercises while in front of a mirror; for example, slightly open and close jaw while supported by your cupped hand.

Massage both sides of the face along the jaw and behind your ears.

Make sure you are taking the proper balance of calcium and magnesium for your gender. Read the section on how to balance Calcium and Magnesium.

Don't chew gum right after injury or while still painful. Maybe you should never chew gum again since it can over extend the jaw.

The good news about TMJ is that it may spontaneously heal once your life is less stressful.

Follow Others: Aging Wisdom from Beatitudes, Nature, Kinfolk

Insomnia and Sleep Problems. Everyone has their own idea of what helps them to sleep well. Some say no caffeine; others recommend a warm cup of coffee, tea or hot chocolate to help relax.

I prefer to consider the things that might cause a person to awaken and then stay awake. Some guidelines for sleeping through the night better:

Have a set bedtime. Prior to 10 pm is recommended because human being's biological clock prepares us for sleep then.

Do not fall asleep on the couch or in front of the TV. When we awaken after 10 pm, it will be harder to get back to sleep.

Take a magnesium supplement along with a light snack (granola or crackers) before going to bed.

At nighttime, set the bedroom temperature cooler than it is set for daytime.

For winter, don't combine flannel sheets and heavy PJs. Mix and match so as not to overheat under the covers, and then catch a chill when you toss off blankets.

If you wake up in the night, get up promptly to empty your bladder, eat some nuts or a cracker (to prevent low blood sugar) and sip some water. If you experience muscle pain, take T-relief/ Traumeel. Get right into bed with lights and electronics off.

Sleep Apnea. This snoring malady gets worse with aging, due to the excessive sag of throat muscles and/or weight gain.

Some tips you may not have tried: Avoid alcoholic beverages, tranquillizers, sleeping pills and anti-histamines before retiring; Sleep prone or on your side; Raise the head of the bed (adjustable bed).

Follow Others: Aging Wisdom from Beatitudes, Nature, Kinfolk

Warning: Snoring interrupted by periods of ten seconds of silence may indicate the snorer lacks for oxygen. He/she will wake themselves up with a snort. See a sleep professional.

Vaccines the Aging Should Consider. Vaccines provide immunity to specific infectious diseases. They all are grown in a medium, use a delivery system, and carry a specific response trigger. People can have an allergic response to any of these three parts. Advise medical staff of any known allergies. NOTE: Younger and/or athletic men and women experience bicep pain at an injection site. Ibuprofen or Tylenol will reduce inflammation.

Pneumonia—This infection of the lungs due to a cold or the flu, is responsible for the deaths of many seniors. For this reason doctors recommend that those individuals over sixty get two pneumonia vaccinations with a one year interval between each.

CAUTION: Everyone should check side effects for any drug they are taking. For example, Lisinopril is commonly given to lower blood pressure. Pneumonia is one of its known side effects in women over 60 who take this drug. In another section in this book, read about taking Beet powder as an option.

Flu Vaccine—Seniors if retired should decide if exposure to the flu is likely. Those still working with the public, may be required to take this vaccine. The flu could lead to infections that are dangerous for seniors. The Covid19 flu vaccine is available to seniors.Strategies for fighting the flu and Covid19:

Follow Others: Aging Wisdom from Beatitudes, Nature, Kinfolk

Oscillococcium is a homeopathic remedy for the flu. Take one entire tube (from 3-tube pack) at first flu symptoms. Go to bed, drink warm liquids and sleep.

Tamiflu is a flu remedy for someone who did not take the flu shot. It requires a doctor's prescription. If a member of your household is given this prescription, all members of the house must take it. Otherwise, high fevers may result.

Zinc, available in a homeopathic dissolvable tablet, has proven useful in fighting Covid19 flu.

Shingles Vaccine—Shingles is a senior's version of the chicken pox. You must have had the juvenile version in order to contract shingles. Shingles break out along a nerve path most often on the mid-section or the forehead. The rash may itch or just be painful. Points to consider:

You can catch shingles if around school children with chicken pox or from someone who just received the live shingles vaccine.

You can catch shingles more than once.

Take vitamin B-12 to reduce and/or eliminate most of the rash and or pain associated with shingles.

Some symptoms of aging discussed above can be experienced at any age. If preventative measures are not taken, aging disease will begin to manifest. A doctor recently told my spouse at his physical that he is older yet healthier than the doctor himself, who has to take four medicines.

We take vitamin supplements at our house and among my family. I sometimes joke that my body is my condominium unit, because I have

Follow Others: Aging Wisdom from Beatitudes, Nature, Kinfolk

spent at least that amount of money on supplementation since 1978. Recently a health-related article stated that it is not uncommon for a person to spend as much as $100K to maintain health and beauty while aging. I guess my supplement "habit" is not as unique as I thought.

Doctor Shaklee's Vitamin Cure

One day Robert Shaklee realized his second son, Forrest, would never become a farmer. So he spent time to encourage young Forrest's mind through books, acquaintances and Chautauqua programs. At one of these popular events, they watched and listened as William Jennings Bryan spoke. A lawyer and statesman, he was among the best known individuals in America. Forrest was impressed with his gestures; he would copy Bryan's stance with raised hands when a speaker himself.

In 1914, Forrest enrolled at the Palmer School of Chiropractic in Davenport, Iowa, to begin a medical career. He disagreed with B.J. Palmer's opinion that only chiropractic should be used to treat patients. Forrest knew first hand that good nutrition played a significant role in health. In Davenport he met two well-known speakers who further influenced his thoughts: Elbert Hubbard, a writer and philosopher, and Clarence Darrow, the popular lawyer.

The positive attitude and powers of persuasion learned stood Forrest in good stead when he applied for a loan at a national bank. He needed capital to purchase equipment for his office. He told the manager that three dollars was all he had except for what was stored in his head; he got the loan. When Forrest began his new practice in 1915 in Rockwell City, Iowa, he recommended nutrition along with chiropractic procedures for his patients.

History with Vitamins. Forrest Shaklee had compounded his Vitalized Minerals at the same time as Polish biochemist, Casimir Funk. Both men recognized that nutrition could help prevent deficiency disorders. (Read the section How Vitamins Got Their Name.)

Dr. Shaklee had begun treatment based on X-ray results before proper safety techniques were known. In 1921 he developed open lesions on his shoulder and leg. A doctor diagnosed those spots as cancerous, caused from X-ray exposure. Shaklee refused the recommended amputations, closed his clinic, went home to Iowa and spent the next three years with only nutrition, rest and Nature to treat himself. After six months the lesions slowly began to heal. He had survived tuberculosis as an infant by natural means; he would survive cancer by the same methods.

A healed Shaklee opened another clinic which completely burned down in 1929. To keep himself and his former patients supplied with Vitalized Minerals and other nutritional supplements, Forrest and his two young boys spent hours stuffing these compounds into capsules and tamping them down.

In 1956, Shaklee interested his two grown sons in production of nutritional supplements for sale nationally. Business-savvy, they opted for distribution by a sales force motivated through bonuses and recognition. With the help of their wives, distributors were signed up to sell Shaklee products to friends and family.

As founder of the company now known worldwide, Dr. Forrest C. Shaklee had built the business around a simple set of values. He wanted to create nutritional and eco-friendly products, not only effective but as pure as possible. Dr. Shaklee survived TB and cancer to live until 93.

[Author has taken Shaklee vitamin and supplements since 1978. Her distributor contact link: https://pws.shaklee.com/donnaaford]

Follow Others: Aging Wisdom from Beatitudes, Nature, Kinfolk

End Point: A new vitamin offering is a customized selection of vitamins and herbs in packets delivered to your home. The customized choices are based on questions you have to answer.

Reputable vitamin companies, like Shaklee, have for a long time offered packets of vitamin essentials based on gender and age. The contents of these packets are determined by advanced clinical studies.

A more recent delivery system for supplements is in carrier solutions, made of liposomes, that quickly deliver large molecule product within the body. Seniors should be careful to take smaller doses with this delivery system in order to prevent irritation of mucosal tissue.

Prayer Point: "Our current age is the result of what we have and have not done up to this point in life." Unknown

Follow Others: Aging Wisdom from Beatitudes, Nature, Kinfolk

Follow Others: Aging Wisdom from Beatitudes, Nature, Kinfolk

Beatitude: Blessed—enjoying enviable happiness, spiritually prosperous [that is, with life-joy and satisfaction in God's favor and salvation, regardless of their outward conditions]—are the makers and maintainers of peace, for they shall be called the sons of God! Matthew 5:9 Amplified

Chapter 8—Avoid Aging Diseases

We are more than skin deep, so aging doesn't stop there. We're made up of bones, blood vessels, fat, brain cells and major organs. All of these age at a rate similar to our skin, but this is not necessarily the same as our biological/natural age. That's where good nutrition, exercise and mental attitude make the difference.

Chronic pain is no joke. Life becomes limited if we can't move around independently because of chronic back, hip or knee pain. I always blame pain on my physical environment first. I've been called "Princess Pea" after a fable. A prince chose for his wife the girl who could detect a pea buried under heaped up mattresses and bedding. That would have been me!

Bones/Joints

Arthritis. The enemy of joints has earned the generic name of Arthritis. Osteoarthritis is caused by excessive wear and tear on overused joints. Another type, Rheumatoid arthritis, is an autoimmune condition that causes inflammation of joint linings. Regardless of the cause, injured joints swell and cause pain while engaged in normal activities.

Joints are what make us flexible, so creaking or sore problems areas due to aging can be: Hips, Knees; Shoulders, Arms; Neck and Back; Hands, wrists, fingers.

Follow Others: Aging Wisdom from Beatitudes, Nature, Kinfolk

Specific suggestions follow in this chapter. Here are some generic tips to try as well: Healthy diets; Moderate exercise, such as walking; Be leery of doctor-prescribed anti-inflammatory NSAIDS that have side-effects; Give up resentful thoughts which encourage arthritis.

Read the sections on Natural Healers and Ointments/Treatments in Chapter 12. Read Pain Management in Chapter 14.

Hips. A researcher on hips claims that the correct position for human posture is that of a pregnant woman. She says that a sucked in abdomen and stuck out chest is about the worst posture for healthy hips. Unfortunately, that is what we've been told to do.

She also claims that hip surgery is useless for prevention for on-going hip pain. My ex-husband has already had three hip surgeries. Her book and CD demonstrate the exercises to fix annoying hip pain before surgery is required. Might be worth checking before you schedule a visit with the surgeon. I do some of the exercises every morning when I get out of bed and daily in my shower. See my fall story later in this chapter.

Minimize hip pain:

Wear a low arch in a shoe. The heel height should be flat or an inch high.

Add a lift to one or both of your heals; get custom orthotics if one leg is longer than the other.

Check the section on orthopedic buying concerns before purchasing beds, chairs and car seats.

Get a firm cushion for any chair that doesn't fit well. You hips and knees should be on the same level. This is an ergonomic recommendation; review other recommendations online.

Follow Others: Aging Wisdom from Beatitudes, Nature, Kinfolk

Check for bursitis. If a cortisone shot eliminates the pain, even temporarily, you know it is inflamed tissue around the joint and not bone-related.

Excessive weight-lifting exercises done while younger can damage hips so that hip replacement surgery may be required. Consult a doctor.

Excessive tightening of the hip muscles, create a bone-on bone condition. Stretching exercises may help.

Femur Necrosis, a type of osteoporosis that weakens the femur bone making it porous.

Osteoporosis. Both genders can experience bone loss when aging bones no longer repair themselves. Women are more susceptible after menopause when estrogen no longer is available to protect against this condition. Bone loss may occur in various areas of the body such as the neck, forearm, spine and hips. Doctors will check for bone-loss with a DEXA scan in post-menopausal women and elderly men. This type of bone loss looks like tunnels through the bone.

Calcium and Magnesium are both needed to prevent osteoporosis. Read the section in chapter 9 on the balance needed for Calcium-Magnesium dependent on gender.

Vitamin D and Boron are also recommended for calcium absorption.

Weight-lifting exercises put stress on hip joints, making them susceptible to arthritis and fracture.

Load-bearing exercises such as walking are excellent prevention strategies to avoid this condition. Wear shoes with laces or Velcro closure to keep ankles in place over rough terrain.

Limit alcoholic beverages and use of corticosteroids.

Follow Others: Aging Wisdom from Beatitudes, Nature, Kinfolk

There are drugs that doctors can recommend to delay bone loss. If the X-rays spot osteoporosis in your hips, doctors will warn that a fall may cause broken bones. For this scenario, infusions of an osteoporosis medication will be recommended. As soon as osteoporosis is suspected, try some of the tips listed above to avoid these consequences.

Shoulder and Knee Injuries. Repetitive stresses to joints, such as the shoulder or knee, can damage tendons that support the joints. Falls and bone spurs can also injure these joints. At the office of the orthopedic doctor who performed my shoulder surgery, the waiting room was literally filled with seniors who had or were about to have knee or shoulder surgery.

Shoulder injuries can result from a fall, repetitive use or overhead/ heavy lifting. Also bone spurs (see below) can cause tears in the rotator cuff. Severe injuries require surgical repair followed by weeks of shoulder therapy, massage and continued exercises with pulleys and rubber bands. Without proper exercise, the shoulder may "freeze" or be unable to be raised up in front or behind the body.

Knee injuries, likewise, result from a fall or repetitive use. A twisting motion that over extends the knee can also cause injury. Cortisone shots and knee supports are the doctor's first remedy. If relief is only temporary, surgical repair followed by weeks of knee therapy may be next. Don't overdo therapy; it can damage the hip muscles.

Tips before surgery: Exercises for the knee are mandatory after surgery, so why not try some therapy and/or exercise prior to surgery. Biofreeze products may allow gentle exercise. CAUTION: Stop if pain becomes worse; any therapy or exercise that causes severe pain indicates the need for an MRI; Stretching may help reposition tight hips before surgery.

Follow Others: Aging Wisdom from Beatitudes, Nature, Kinfolk

Tips after surgery: Homeopathic remedy, Arnica Montana 30c, should be taken whenever pain is experienced. Pain after injury or surgery usually signals healing. Arnica assists with the healing process and thus relieves the immediate pain of that process; Take Arnica Montana 200c to wean yourself off of post-surgery pain medication as soon as possible; Wait to start therapy until advised by your surgeon; Set new goals for yourself within the bounds recommended by your surgeon.

Bone Spurs. Spurs are pointy growths of calcium that often occur in shoulders and on feet. Although the growth itself is made up of calcium, the excretion of calcium is related to low magnesium. Read the section on how to balance Calcium and Magnesium.

A mailman with a bone spur on his ankle had the surgery to remove the spur. It returned until he took the proper ratio of calcium/magnesium.

Healing Back and Neck Surgeries. Trauma to any portion of the neck or spinal column can require surgery in order to fix. Early surgeries of this type required using cadaver or the patient's own bone to surround the injured and stabilize it until new bone growth appeared in twelve weeks. Bed rest and neck or back brace was used to immobilize the area. Nowadays screws are inserted to stabilize; however, recovery time remains the same while waiting for bone growth to occur.

Doctors are less apt to suggest surgery to older patients. Steroids and cortisone shots are recommended instead.

My back surgery was due to a pinched ganglion (bundle of nerves) near my lower spine. The immediate cause of the back injury was lifting an engine-puller component that was too heavy. It was also aggravated by driving a standard car with a shift stick set too high for my short-waist body type.

Follow Others: Aging Wisdom from Beatitudes, Nature, Kinfolk

When a surgeon cuts into the spinal area, he also cuts muscle. Now, there are two areas that require healing: the injured spine area and the muscle groups that were cut. My surgeon promised that the ganglion pain would be gone almost immediately. His prediction was accurate. He also promised that all the pain would eventually go away. The muscle healing, however, took eight months. Stretching my spine against a wall or on the floor was the only thing that stopped muscle spasms.

Tips to speed the healing: Take Arnica Montana, 200c for weeks after surgery, then 30c if bothered by future pain; Take 1 capsule of Fish Oil daily. This coats the myelin sheath to reduce spinal pain once able to perform tasks like raking leaves.

"Are not two sparrows sold for a farthing? And one of them shall not fall on the ground without your Father." Matthew 10:29

Broken Bones from Falls. Everyone worries at some point about what disease or accident may cause their death. We've heard stories about the older woman who falls and breaks her hip, then never makes it out of the nursing home. Or we know people who received the diagnosis of cancer they always dreaded. Our friend Job in the Bible puts it this way, "For the thing which I greatly feared is come upon me, and that which I was afraid of is come unto me."

My Fall Story. I had no intention of writing this chapter. Other people fall and break bones but not me. When it happened in April 2019, I was sure it was only a sprain, so refused to go to the hospital. Until I had to go down stairs on my butt because I could no longer stand unaided. You guessed it.

When I tripped and fell hard onto the floor, it fractured the head of my femur. Not just any bone mind you; nope, the largest bone in the body.

Follow Others: Aging Wisdom from Beatitudes, Nature, Kinfolk

Note that this story follows Peter's beatitude about obedience; my fall was related to disobeying guidance.

So where am I now? I am at three months into the healing process (total of six months to fully stabilize). I can walk without a cane or walker most of the time, but probably shouldn't when there is danger of falling again. Rough terrain or raised edges of rugs, rising after sitting for a long time, in public settings where I could be bumped or shoved by accident. Falling a second time at this stage is frowned upon.

UPDATE: I had the screws and pins removed after five months. The inflammation caused total separation of the unhealed femur. I am now recovered from a total hip replacement done at nine months.

What I have learned— bone healing is not for the faint hearted.

Building Bones. To rebuild bone your body knows you need to rest, for hours in total sleep, not watching TV or reading. It will raise your blood pressure numbers, may even cause you to pass out, until you comply. Balancing Calcium and Magnesium is a whole new game. Bone aches and muscle cramps may indicate need for extra calcium. Eye twitches mean that you may be getting low on magnesium. Load up your refrigerator with yogurt snacks. Cut back on sugar.

Holding Fluid. You're getting less exercise and potassium levels may be off. Immediately after hip surgery you need to make frequent nighttime trips to the bathroom. Wear Depends or have a port-a-potty close by the bed.

Sleeping positions. Side sleepers may aggravate their good hip. Place small or soft pillow between knees. Bed should be equipped with pull bars to rise after sleeping.

Exercise positions. Walking and moving the legs 20-30 times each is the best exercise. Keep both knees pointed in the same direction. Do

Follow Others: Aging Wisdom from Beatitudes, Nature, Kinfolk

not force right angle bends—not in the waist line or in the knee. Get yourself some pickup tools; once you can reach to the floor, careful stretching is good for your back.

Notice that the leg of a broken femur with pins points outward to protect your hip from fracturing) and is shorter than the other. After total hip replacement, both legs should be the same length and point same way. Screws used to draw the femur bone up to the head, can back out and hurt your leg, especially if hips are not well-padded.

Learn how to play musical chairs and shoes to relieve the throbbing caused by being out of alignment in the spine, hips or legs. Rest on a stool pulled up to a counter top while cooking supper. If pain persists after six months, get another diagnosis. Older women often have poor blood circulation at the femur, so pinning may never heal.

Orthopedic Buyer concerns. Here are some of my suggestions to consider before buying something that may cause you discomfort.

Senior-Friendly Car. Is the new car going to cause pain? Here is a list of things to check before purchasing a car. Don't even consider whether this will be "the last car you ever buy"! That's a true sign of being OLD.

Knees should be same height as the back of the car seat (level and 90 deg angle). Can it be adjusted, or a slanted pillow added?

Steering wheel should be adjusted so arms are kept low when correctly placed on the wheel. Wheel should not hit your knees.

Lumbar support at rear of seat cushion corrects posture; small pillow can do the same.

Follow Others: Aging Wisdom from Beatitudes, Nature, Kinfolk

Automatic transmission is always preferable. If Standard, make sure of two things:

A stick shift is not too high or low to reach easily.

The clutch pedal has any easy throw without excessive stretching or force.

If short or have a short-waist, consider that all crash dummies have long-waists.

Double-check first four points; if adjustments can't be made, choose another car/model/manufacturer. Yes; it's that important.

Senior-Friendly Chair/Recliner. Getting a recliner is almost a badge for those close to retirement age or retired already. And equally it almost guarantees back and hip pain. Here are two reasons why:

Soft, squishy cushions (provide no support)

Reclining position (hips lower than knees most of the time)

In her book Save Your Hips, Christine Kent offers the opinion that the disease called osteoarthritis of the hip is seen in both young athletes and the older adult population. While one type may result from excessive physical training and activity, the other seems rooted in years of poor posture while driving cars and sitting on upholstered furniture. The book comes with a DVD of exercises to help put the hips in their correct relationship with the body.

Instead of a recliner here are some suggestions for best seating choices (important since retirees have more time they can spend seated).

Choose an upright chair with limited padding in the seat and back areas. If knees are not level with back of seat, do one of the following:

Follow Others: Aging Wisdom from Beatitudes, Nature, Kinfolk

Lift the chair's rear legs.

Add a firm pillow (not memory foam), slanted if possible.

If the chair doesn't have lumbar support, position a small decorative pillow between the chair and your spine.

If the chair has arms, make sure their height doesn't cause shoulder pain. Add pillows to adjust.

Limit slouching and/or using a foot stool to recline.

Senior-Friendly Mattress/Pillow. The trick to the perfect mattress is pairing it with the perfect pillow. All mattresses take a set in the area of our seat/hips. This eventually places the body at a downhill incline from head to butt. You can reduce the angle of incline by experimenting with a combination of neck pillows, thin or thick. They should adequately support the neck while reducing the incline. This pillow advice came directly from a neurosurgeon (the one who labeled me geriatric by my age).

Of course, the best pillow is relative to your mattress type, so:

If you just bought a super firm memory foam mattress, remove your shoes and try walking barefoot on top of the mattress. This hint comes from a mattress owner who was actually advised to try this to make their expensive new mattress a bit more comfortable. Make it a family affair, but no bouncing please! As my father often warned: "No horseplay in the house."

If you are searching for a firm mattress, avoid those with memory foam in the butt area. Better to get a well-padded topper if you sleep on your side. I can personally vouch for the fact that memory foam will take a set where you need firmness the most. Try to imagine if the steepness

Follow Others: Aging Wisdom from Beatitudes, Nature, Kinfolk

of the angle from head to butt and then to feet will cause a dip in the butt area.

For more support in the middle of a Queen-sized mattress, order the double box spring option. The mattress will remain firm longer and two small box springs are easier to move on the stairs.

Pillow Talk from Walter. Based on years of experience working in a mattress store, my son-in-law offered this advice for choosing pillows:

Side sleepers need a pillow that is thick enough to accommodate broad or narrow shoulders.

Back and stomach sleepers should choose a flat pillow.

If you are prone to sweating, choose a pillow type that wicks away moisture.

If you move around a lot during the night, you may need more than one pillow.

After hip surgery, side sleepers need a small pillow between legs.

Follow Others: Aging Wisdom from Beatitudes, Nature, Kinfolk

Targeted Food/Supplement – Generic Table

Targeted Food/Supplement – Generic Table

Type	Name	Issue Addressed	Usage
Food/Drink	Cherry Juice	Gout	As needed
	Red meat	Gout	Limit
	Water	Gout	Keep hydrated
	Protein drink	Incontinence	Daily
	Alcohol	Cancer	Eliminate from diet
Vitamin/Mineral	B-3, B-6	Hemorrhoids	
	B-6	Skin Cancer	
	D3	Skipped heart beat	Regulate heart electrical system
	Probiotics	Yeast Infection - bowel	
	Lecithin	Balding/ Cholesterol	Capsule daily
	Fish Oil	Cholesterol	Capsule daily
	Kelp	Thyroid	Tablet or seaweed daily
	Resveratrol	Vision; hormones	
	Selenium	Autoimmune	
Herbs/Tincture	Stone Root	Hemorrhoids	Drops as needed
	Beet Root	High blood pressure	
	Hawthorn Root	High blood pressure	
	Olive Leaf Extract	High blood pressure	
	Milk Thistle	Liver	
Exercise	Kegel	Incontinence	

End Point: For aging diseases specific to males or females, read the chapter that follows.

Prayer Point: Beatitude according to Luke—Blessed are ye when men shall hate you, and when they shall separate you from their company, and shall reproach you, and cast out your name as evil, for the Son of Man's sake. Rejoice ye in that day and leap for joy: for behold your reward is great in heaven; for in like manner did their fathers unto the prophets . Luke 6:22

Follow Others: Aging Wisdom from Beatitudes, Nature, Kinfolk

Beatitude: Blessed and happy and enviably fortunate, and spiritually prosperous [that is, in the state in which one enjoys and finds satisfaction in God's favor and salvation regardless of his outward conditions]—are those who are persecuted for righteousness sake (for being and doing right), for theirs is the kingdom of heaven! Matthew 5:10 Amplified

Chapter 9—Aging By Gender

"But they that wait upon the LORD shall renew their strength; they shall mount up with wings as eagles; they shall run, and not be weary; and they shall walk, and not faint." Isaiah 40:31

Some of us will begin to age earlier than others, most likely due to genetics. Except for accidental death (or the rapture), we will all experience at least a few of the issues mentioned in this chapter.

Was there a time in your life when you could lift, push or move anything? The muscles in a man's arms are capable of great force. Whereas a woman's leg muscles are her natural strength. How sad to hold up an arm or leg and notice the skin sag to reveal 'millions' of tiny wrinkles where there was once smooth skin. That's when I found it hardest to obey the tenth commandment, "Thou shalt not covet thy neighbor's" [smooth skin, muscles, etc.], Exodus 20:17.

By Gender. Time to talk about aging issues that specifically affect females vs. males, and vice versa. At the end of each section there is a list of targeted natural remedies to try. The emphasis is on prevention using natural remedies, not necessarily a cure. Always consult a physician with questions regarding your health.

Are Natural Remedies Effective? As mentioned earlier in this book, I began studying nutrition, healthy eating and natural remedies in the

Follow Others: Aging Wisdom from Beatitudes, Nature, Kinfolk

1970s. I remember people fearing that the government would ban vitamins; it never happened. Believe me, if these remedies were not effective, they would be long gone from our shelves. Certainly, no one, like myself, would have continued taking them for almost fifty years.

Are Natural Remedies Safe? Doctors and news articles frequently issue warnings about taking vitamins and herbs. In general any side effects are minor and easily fixed when you stop taking the remedy. However, when scheduled for surgery, you will receive a list of remedies to stop taking a week or more before the date of surgery. This doesn't mean they are unsafe. Doctor concerns are related to possible bleeding side effects. Also, it is their responsibility to protect your life.

WARNING: Always follow pre-op requests.

This chapter and the previous offer some natural solutions to consider trying when your doctor's care is for routine health issues. Be sure to follow the guidelines below for taking a new remedy.

Steps to Introduce a new remedy (same as introduction for chapter 7)

WARNING: If you are under doctor's care for any condition, discuss the content of this document with that professional. Medications may need to be adjusted as your health improves.

IMPORTANT: It is always best to consult with a doctor or medical professional to get a proper diagnosis. If the medicine prescribed does not work for you, that is the point when you may decide to try one of the natural remedies mentioned in this chapter. Follow the steps recommended below (in fact, this is similar to the appropriate procedure to try any new pharmaceutical medication):

Take the prescribed dosage per the bottle. If it makes you feel ill, stop immediately. Otherwise, try for two weeks.

Follow Others: Aging Wisdom from Beatitudes, Nature, Kinfolk

If the issue has gotten worse, stop at the 2-week mark. Blame everything from pimples to constipation on the remedy. If your issue is improved or at least not gotten worse, continue for two more weeks.

If there is no improvement at one month, stop the remedy. Go to next step. If nothing worse and maybe better, continue taking for 2 more weeks.

At six weeks, add this to your regular regimen if improvement is noticed. If results are not obvious, stop and re-evaluate in a month; you may have missed some positive change.

Female Issues

"Despise not thy mother when she is old" Proverbs 23:22

Menopause Issues. Like puberty, menopause is a time of life when levels of hormones change. These changes, similar to those that occur when pregnant, can cause issues for night sweats to tears, bladder leakage when you cough or sneeze, etc. All that fun stuff we call menopause. Some women will experience fewer menopause issues than others, at an earlier or later age. What happens endocrine-wise, is that due to decreased levels of estrogen, one of the other hormones, (thyroid, adrenal, pituitary) must pick up the slack from the female glands. Read Dr. Abravanel's diet based on strongest gland in chapter 11. Post menopause, the adrenal glands pick up the entire slack; this results in all aging women having belly fat and loss of hour glass shape.

Excessive Menstrual Blood Flow. Consult a gynecologist: Severe bleeding from the uterus can quickly turn into hemorrhaging. Always contact a medical professional if you fill a sanitary pad in less than 20 minutes! This may require a D&C procedure done in the doctor's office.

Follow Others: Aging Wisdom from Beatitudes, Nature, Kinfolk

Hot flashes. Not dangerous but equally stressful, are the hot flashes that many women experience around this time of life. Fortunately, I never had a single hot flash. I credit this to the Soy Protein shakes I took morning and evening along with my vitamins. Soy affects the thyroid and can lower body temperature. Later, I had to switch to whey or pea-protein based drinks to raise my body temperature a full degree to counteract the cold hands and feet my blood pressure beta blocker constantly causes. The homeopathic remedy, Lachesis Mutus, may help with hot flashes. See table below.

Dry Vagina. A woman's sex life may diminish with age, but I can vouch that it need not go away. However, a dry vagina from reduced hormones in the body can make the act uncomfortable for both partners. You can use a liquid Glide technology. Or you can take a single pill a day to relieve the problem. GLA comes from borage oil, a hormone-like substance in a capsule taken orally that results in just the right amount of natural hormone-inspired lubrication. Shaklee sells the GLA product that I take. This works similar to Primrose Oil capsules, which not everyone can tolerate. In your seventies you may need to add a hormone cream; see your female doctor.

Iron Storage Disease – Consult a doctor: Both men and women can have iron storage disease. Men must donate blood all their lives in order to keep their iron levels under control. Storage of excessive iron will cause the person to become extremely tired. This is one time women can say that menstruation is useful; they only experience the extreme tiredness prior to puberty and then post menopause.

IMPORTANT: For both sexes, always verify that your multiple vitamin does not contain iron or large amounts of vitamin C (required to absorb iron). This means you should avoid any multiple that is labeled as a Women's vitamin supplement; always take the Men's version. Read Vitamin Basics.

Follow Others: Aging Wisdom from Beatitudes, Nature, Kinfolk

Bowel/Bladder Issues.

Gravity plays an important role in aging. Muscle groups sag and core exercises, such as presented in pool or Tai Chi exercises are vitally important. Tightening CORE muscles can improve posture and breathing, as well.

Bladder Leakage/ Incontinence. Women may think we are the only sex with issues of bladder leakage—when we cough, sneeze and later as we exercise and even move about. Depends protection comes in sizes, shapes and colors to fit all of us aged folk. These do offer mobility.

Or try some of these solutions that you may not know about:

Protein is as necessary to maintain CORE muscles as it is for biceps. I've taken a protein drink daily since 1978 just for this reason.

Squat when you feel a sneeze coming; this causes the upper thigh muscles to tighten. This can prevent leakage, although you might feel a bit conspicuous about doing a squat in a public space.

Kegel exercises tighten the pelvic floor muscles as well as the opening to the urethra. You can practice inconspicuously in the car, at your computer and at home. Doctors suggest you do not practice the Kegel maneuver to stop normal urine flow, as this could interfere with the ability to empty the bladder. My suggestion is do not practice excessively because, like any other muscle, thigh muscles could cramp on you.

Squeeze a roll of bathroom tissue between your legs to tighten the target muscles.

Bladder Infection – Consult a doctor immediately. Bladder infections are notorious to the aged, frequently after hospital visits. A MRSA bladder infection can cause hallucinations. Due to the ability to hide out

Follow Others: Aging Wisdom from Beatitudes, Nature, Kinfolk

internally, MRSA is difficult to eliminate. IMPORTANT: this type of Urinary Tract Infection (UTI) must be treated ASAP with strong antibiotics.

Suggestions for natural treatments you can try to ward off a UTI:

Homeopathic remedy, Cantharis, may help prevent UTIs. See table below. Take immediately whenever trips to the bathroom are more frequent or painful than usual.

Drink cranberry juice; increase your vitamin C intake.

Hemorrhoids. Hemorrhoids that protrude or bleed are stressful, more so, they could become life threatening. Constipation and heavy lifting may trigger incidences of bleeding. Long rides and soft seats can make matters worse. IMPORTANT: Consult a physician to be sure that any bleeding from the bowel area is not related to cancer.

A rectal doctor can perform in-office procedures, such as an elastic band to cutoff blood flow from an external hemorrhoid. Stubborn cases with excessive blood flow may require surgery. Things to consider before hemorrhoid surgery:

Assume a knees-up, V-shaped position on the toilet, so gravity can assist with bowel movements. If you are short, purchase a foot stool designed to help keep your legs at the right angle.

Wear pants that do not fit tightly around the waist; wear underwear without raised internal seams.

Consider a stool softener, add fiber to diet or take a laxative as a temporary solution.

Add a B-complex or brewer's yeast tablet containing B-3 and B-6 vitamins to your regimen for long-term solution.

Follow Others: Aging Wisdom from Beatitudes, Nature, Kinfolk

Remedies to reduce symptoms:

Use witch hazel (an ingredient in hemorrhoid ointments) as a wipe for bloody discharges to reduce inflammation.

Stone Root is an herb that helps regulate circulation in the extremities. For persistent symptoms, place several drops of Stone Root tincture in water covering the bottom of the glass. Place in your mouth and hold for a minute or two, before swallowing.

Insert a 400 mg Vitamin E capsule into the bowel while lying prone. Resist the urge to evacuate to let the capsule dissolve. Vitamin E heals scar tissue.

Yeast Infection. Candidiasis is a fungal disease which can take over bacterial colonies in mucus-lined tissues such as found in the vagina and intestine. Normally found in the body, if antibiotics allow this yeast to thrive in the intestine, it changes into a fungus with tentacles able to pierce intestinal walls. It can then travel through the body and manifest as immune system issues especially food allergies.

Probiotics are advised along with lengthy abstinence of yeast favorite foods, such as bread and carbohydrates. Yogurt helps the body create its own probiotics. Plain yogurt is best to eat with cereal, oatmeal and as a snack with applesauce.

Also read the section Prebiotics and Cultured Foods in Chapter 10.

Natural Tips for Yeast Infection: Yeast-killing medications can be prescribed as a treatment by a doctor, applied topically or taken orally. Watch for allergic reactions, such as increased redness of the skin; Douche with vinegar (available at drug store) or with plain yogurt; Wear cotton underwear, white preferably. Some colored underwear have white panel linings. Allow times to air dry, if discomfort is extreme.

Follow Others: Aging Wisdom from Beatitudes, Nature, Kinfolk

Breast Cancer – Consult a doctor immediately. One of the first nutritional facts I learned was from a *biochemist. I have forgotten his name, but not his recommendations about breast cancer prevention.

Tips for natural prevention strategies that few know: Take a tablet of the mineral Manganese daily, even if your multiple has this nutrient. Manganese protects breast tissue; Eat sunflower and pumpkin seeds daily. These foods are sources for manganese.

I also make *his delicious Eggplant Soup recipe regularly every fall - forty years later.

Ovarian Cancer – Consult a doctor immediately. We each have a cause that is dear to our hearts. Two years ago, Ovarian cancer became a personal war for me. A dear friend died within one year (twelve months) after diagnosis. The symptoms were a swollen abdomen and lack of appetite. Could have been anything; it was ovarian cancer and alcohol usage made it a fatal disease.

Another friend's friend got the same diagnosis at that time, but she still had her uterus—blood post menopause was her first symptom. Both women, like actress Audrey Hepburn, died within months of the diagnosis. Why? Diagnosis isn't given until ovarian cancer is at stage 3 or 4, when the patient has 1% chance of living a year. There are no early warning screens, like for breast cancer.

Tumors form inside the abdominal lining, with one large one that doctor's will use chemo to shrink before surgery. Unfortunately, once the largest tumor is removed, hundreds of microscopic cancers (like grains of sands) that remain will grow. These can entwine the bowel and shut down digestion. Only a G-tube installation and limited diet can keep the patient alive. Not the quality of life most of us desire.

Follow Others: Aging Wisdom from Beatitudes, Nature, Kinfolk

To be safe: Get checkups regularly, whether or not you still have uterus, ovaries, breasts and appendix.

Have the test to see if you are prone to tumor growth. If you and your daughters have this trait, you will be asked to consider removal of your female organs.

Don't drink alcohol of any kind and frequency. Women are notoriously unable to handle alcohol as well as men do. More specifically, the liver must be clean in order to handle all the toxins that chemotherapy treatments will dump into the body.

Talk to your doctor about immunotherapy instead of chemotherapy. This leaves a portion of the largest tumor to discourage growth of smaller tumors. Keytruda is a immunotherapy medication targeted to lung cancer. Research any new therapy thoroughly before surgery.

When declared cancer free, DO NOT celebrate with liquor. Protect your liver and ask for continued prayer instead. IMPORTANT: Toxicity due to dying cells can be deadly. Wow! Sad truths.

Follow Others: Aging Wisdom from Beatitudes, Nature, Kinfolk
Targeted Food/Supplement Table – Female Issues

Targeted Food/Supplement Table - Female Issues

Type	Name	Issue Addressed	Usage
Food/Drink	Sunflower Seeds/ Pumpkin Seeds – raw	Breast health	Daily
	Yogurt	Yeast infection - bowel	Daily
	Protein drink	Bladder leakage	Daily
	Alcohol	Ovarian Cancer	Eliminate from diet
	Soy protein/flour	Hot Flashes - Menopause	Daily
	Cranberry juice	UTI	At sign of infection
Vitamin/Mineral (above multiple)	Manganese	Breast health	Daily
	GLA	Dry vagina - menopause	Daily
	Probiotics	Yeast Infection - bowel	Daily
	Vitamin B-3, B-6	Hemorrhoids	Brewer's Yeast
	Vitamin B-6	Skin Cancer	Daily
	Vitamin B-12	Anemia	Low-potency sublingual tablet
	Vitamin C	UTI	Increase dosage
	Resveratrol	Youth; hormones	
	Multiple w/o Iron & C	Iron Storage disease	Take a multiple; no iron and extra C
Herb/Tincture	Stone Root	Hemorrhoids	Drops as needed
Homeopathic	Cantharis	Bladder Infection	30c, as needed
	Lachesis Mutus	Hot Flashes - Menopause	30c, as needed
Exercise	Kegel	Bladder leakage	Schedule exercise 2x week

Follow Others: Aging Wisdom from Beatitudes, Nature, Kinfolk
Male Issues From Head to Toe

"Beauty of old men is the grey head." Proverbs 20:29

Balding/Gray Hair. Funny that we start with the hair of aged men. Forehead balding is one of the first indicators that a man is aging. Later, he will develop the distinguished gray sideburns. Male-pattern baldness slowly proceeds from forehead baldness to reveal the shiny top/front of his head. I think bald looks distinguished on a man. Unfortunately, women can also develop male-pattern baldness.

Tips to slow the aging of hair/scalp: Soy Lecithin – take daily in capsule or granular forms to slow down the balding process; Folic acid – take at least 800 mcg of this B-vitamin daily to help reduce the amount of hair turning gray. FYI, hair grays when the root bulbs no longer have color; After hair turns gray consider a blue shampoo to reduce hard-water stain on the hair.

Beer Gut. Men have a higher need for B-vitamins (B-1 and B-3) found in brewer's yeast. This may partly explain why they often prefer to drink beer as opposed to wine (women's choice). But what causes that beer belly?

In chapter 11, read about the body-type diet. Fat accumulates on the body based on our preference for trigger foods. Alcohol is one of the trigger foods for the adrenal gland. My strongest gland is the adrenal so body fat has always accumulated on my abdomen. No, I don't ever drink beer or alcohol of any kind. But I do love nuts, cream and butter which are also adrenal triggers.

Gout. Gout typically starts in the large toe. This is a painful joint condition that occurs after consumption of purines found in meat, beer, etc. Sharp, uric acid crystals form at joints. Limit the foods listed below

Follow Others: Aging Wisdom from Beatitudes, Nature, Kinfolk

that are known to trigger gout attacks; kidney stones are also formed by consumption of the same foods:

Red meat and organ meats (liver, tongue and sweetbreads)

Shellfish such as shrimp and lobster

Sugary beverages

Excessive alcohol especially beer (more than one alcoholic drink for women and two for men within 24 hours)

Avoid dehydration

Cherry juice is a natural remedy. Limit how much juice you drink since most of the commercial brands are sweetened with apple juice (high in carbs).

Drink sufficient water; gout crystals form when the body is dehydrated.

Iron Storage Disease. Both men and women are subject to this blood disease. See the section earlier in this chapter for women.

Kidney Stones. Passing a kidney stone is right up there in pain with childbirth. Sharp crystals must pass done through a narrow passage way. My spouse has experienced this twice. Below are tips he uses to avoid having anymore.

Unfiltered water could result in kidney stones, especially if local water has a high ratio of calcium. Stick to bottled water if that is your local scenario. Dehydration is another cause of kidney stones as well as causing gout.

Follow Others: Aging Wisdom from Beatitudes, Nature, Kinfolk

Testosterone Deficiency - Male Menopause. What happens endocrine-wise, is that testosterone production decreases. So one of the other hormones, (thyroid, adrenal, pituitary) must pick up the slack. Read Dr. Abravanel's diet based on strongest gland in chapter 11. Eventually, the adrenal gland picks up the slack; this results in all men having more belly fat.

Erectile Dysfunction. Aging is no joke when it intrudes in the private corners of our lives. No guy expects to experience Erectile Dysfunction (ED), any more than a women in her 30s expects to see wrinkles lines on a once attractive face. Poor health can cause Erectile Dysfunction (ED). Get a yearly physical with blood work that checks for diabetes, heart disease, prostate cancer and kidney disease.

There is a Biblical quote worth noting. Proverbs 2:6 promises "The curse causeless shall not come." When we ignore or abuse our health, aging gains speed in our lives. Reversals are possible, but prevention is the wisest plan. There are a few things to consider.

Blood Pressure meds are known to cause ED. Try some natural suggestions to lower blood pressure given in the previous chapter on Generic Aging. Check any other medications for possible links to ED.

Muscle Loss – Sarcopenia. Are your muscles less able to lift, push or move anything? General suggestions to prevent sarcopenia:

Start or get back to exercise ASAP. Read chapter 12 to choose the best exercise for your body type; also exercises specific for flabby arms.

Include in your daily diet protein drinks (preferably from a mix stirred into a nut milk).

Replace wheat bread with that made with rye flour for less muscle loss.

Follow Others: Aging Wisdom from Beatitudes, Nature, Kinfolk

Bladder Leakage. Men can experience bladder leakage if there is an issue with flow blockage due to the prostate. Bladder leakage will result after surgery for prostate cancer.

Protein is as necessary to maintain CORE muscles as it is for biceps. A protein drink taken daily is recommended for this reason.

Kegel exercises tighten the pelvic floor muscles as well as the mouth of the urethra. These exercises are recommended to men after surgery for prostate. You can practice inconspicuously in the car, at your computer and at home. Doctors suggest you do not practice the Kegel maneuver to stop regular urine flow, as this could interfere with the ability to empty the bladder. My suggestion is do not practice excessively because, like any other muscle, thigh muscles could cramp on you.

Colon Cancer. Men are at greater risk to experience colon cancer. Be sure to get a colonoscopy at least every five years after 50. Take a magnesium supplement; men need some calcium but never more than 50% calcium to 50% magnesium. A sign of being low in magnesium is muscle spasms of the eyelid.

Prostate – Consult a doctor immediately. A urologist told a friend recently that an enlarged prostate gland is as much a sign of aging as is gray hair. A typical symptom is reduced urine flow and frequent need to urinate. High PSA test results can indicate possible issues with the prostate. A urologist can tell for sure.

The doctor will use sonar to determine if the bladder empties fully. A physical exam is the test for a lump on the gland. And you may even need a second PSA blood test to give a reliable set of numbers. Should results indicate, the urologist will then perform a biopsy to check for

Follow Others: Aging Wisdom from Beatitudes, Nature, Kinfolk

cancer cells. If warranted, the doctor will order bone scans to check for possible metastasized cancer.

Flomax – this drug will be prescribed to help the bladder empty fully, especially of concern for diabetics. Diabetes can cause damage to the small blood vessels in the kidneys, so retention of fluid is not acceptable. This is also used in cases of kidney stones.

Saw Palmetto – may be an option for relieving the above symptoms as long as no prostate cancer or diabetes is detected.

Zinc – a slight deficiency of this mineral can lead to enlargement of the prostate. Pumpkin seeds and fruit are natural sources of zinc.

Prostate Cancer Options. If the biopsy reveals the presence of cancer in the prostate only, recommendations are currently based on two factors: age and Gleason grade from biopsy results. Options are some combination of surgery and/or radiation administered with female hormone.

Below 70 years old: surgery is recommended with a second biopsy required at the time of surgery. There is a single operation procedure that enters through the bowel area. There is a two operation procedure that enters from the back side.

Between 70-75: optional decision from one of the other two choices; doctors will push toward radiation treatment.

Between 75-80: Female hormone therapy for nine months to shrink prostate; radiation treatment with various delivery options and number of sessions required. Diarrhea often results from radiation treatment. Eat yogurt or take acidophilus capsules to reduce this side effect.

The cancer surgeon or radiation specialist will explain all the options with pros/cons, including which options are not available based on

Follow Others: Aging Wisdom from Beatitudes, Nature, Kinfolk

individual results. If the cancer has metastasized outside of the prostate wall, other treatments will include female hormones, surgery and chemotherapy.

Targeted Food/Supplement Table – Male Issues

Targeted Food/Supplement Table - Male Issues

Type	Name	Issue Addressed	Usage
Food/Drink	Cherry Juice	Gout	As needed
	Red meat	Gout	Limit
	Water	Gout; Kidney stones	
	Protein drink	Bladder leakage; muscle	Daily
	Alcohol	Cancer	Eliminate from diet
	Rye bread	Muscle tone	Instead of wheat
Vitamin/Mineral (above multiple)	Vitamin B-1, B-3	Beer belly	
	Vitamin B-6	Skin Cancer; hemorrhoids	
	Folic Acid (B vitamin)	Graying hair - reduce	800 mcg daily
	Probiotics	Yeast Infection - bowel	daily
	Lecithin	Balding	Several capsules daily
	Zinc	Prostate health	50 mg daily
	Resveratrol	Youth	
	Multiple w/o Iron & C	Iron Storage disease	Take multiple; no iron and extra C
Herb/Tincture	Stone Root	Hemorrhoids	Drops as needed
	Saw Palmetto	Blocked urine flow	1 capsule 2x daily
	Stinging Nettle	Hair; sexual stimulant	
	Beet Root	ED with high blood pressure	
	Hawthorn Root	ED with high blood pressure	
	Olive Leaf Extract	ED with high blood pressure	
Exercise	Kegel	Bladder leakage	
	Diet specific exercise	Muscle tone	

Chapter 9—Aging By Gender

Follow Others: Aging Wisdom from Beatitudes, Nature, Kinfolk

Achsa Corliss Outlived Three Husbands.

Every family has a member with the spirit of a pioneer—one who dared more than others, lost and gained back repeatedly and never quit trying. Achsa Corliss(1858-1939) was that one in our family.

Born in Vermont prior to the Civil War, Achsa [axe-a] Hutchins married at eighteen and travelled west with her new husband who found employment building railroad lines. He would leave her at their home base in Minnesota for extended periods of time. My granddaughter lives close by that home base, in an area known for winter temperatures of -50 degrees.

Achsa got pregnant three times as her husband returned and left again; she had two miscarriages and one living boy. The father had no idea of his son's age/weight and told a doctor the wrong information. The dosage prescribed caused the boy to become permanently retarded. Kindly women at her home base, took up a collection to send Achsa and her son back to Vermont. She became the first in our family to get a divorce.

For her second marriage my great-grandmother chose a man in his senior years, incorrectly assuming she was less apt to get pregnant. Benjamin Corliss had seen her at a family gathering and told others that she would be his next wife. They married in 1887. Their wedding photograph, which I own, was done with an early salt-peter photographic technique.

Achsa's assumption about the fertility of senior men was wrong. She promptly gave her husband five more children from 1888 to 1897. My grandmother Flora was born in 1893 when her father was seventy-five. Benjamin Corliss died at eighty-nine. Achsa married again in 1915; her third husband, Fred Adams, died in 1927. In Vermont, she spent her last days at the home of her daughter Flossie.

Follow Others: Aging Wisdom from Beatitudes, Nature, Kinfolk

History of the name Achsa. My great-grandmother's first name was Biblical, as were many names given in the 1800s. When the Israelites entered the promised land, only two explorers/spies of the land were still alive: Joshua and Caleb. Both of them believed God and reported back to the Israelites in the desert that they were able to take the land from its occupants. The other ten explorers/spies whined that the inhabitants were giants and would terrify the people. Those who were afraid died in the wilderness as they wished. Joshua and Caleb, still strong warriors in their 80s, marched into the promised land at the head of men forty years their junior.

Caleb's daughter was named Achsa. When she married, her father gave the couple some of his land. She insisted that there also be a water source included in her inheritance. Brave woman—just like our Achsa who outlived three husbands, travelled across early America and passed away peacefully at the age of 81.

Balance Vitamins/Minerals

Calcium and Magnesium Facts. Without calcium in our diet we can break bones. I found that out the hard way two years ago after cracking a rib from excessive coughing in a pneumonia bout. The actual reason was because dairy, which is best source of calcium in our diets, causes congestion. I was trying to exclude these from my diet to get over the incessant cough. Instead, I ended up with a cracked rib due to low calcium.

Without magnesium in our diet we could die of a heart attack even if we jog every day. A well-known doctor and jogging advocate died on a run while in Vermont on vacation. Blood work showed he was low in magnesium which triggered a fatal muscle spasm of the heart.

Follow Others: Aging Wisdom from Beatitudes, Nature, Kinfolk

Why in this day and age is anyone low in magnesium? Because our soil is depleted of this vital nutrient. Foods that should be rich in magnesium are no longer.

IMPORTANT: Muscle spasms of the eyelid indicate low magnesium. Do not ignore since muscle spasms of the heart can be deadly.

Percentages for Optimum Health. Check the label for any supplement you are taking. Men should avoid Female multiple vitamins, and vice versa. Here are the recommended ratios:

All men, young or old, need 50% calcium to 50% magnesium

Women from puberty through menopause need 100% calcium to 50% magnesium

Aging women, post menopause, need 50% calcium to 50% magnesium

Bed Wetting Cure. Another oddity about magnesium is that a lack of it can cause bed wetting in young boys. My sons wet their beds, and my daughter wet herself at school. Their father had been a bed wetter as a boy, too. As soon as I started the family on a calcium-magnesium chewables, all three boys and my daughter stopped wetting at the same time and never did it again. They may all have smaller bladders or higher need for magnesium.

Potassium and Sodium Facts. Cell walls are permeable to permit flow of nutrients into the cell and to remove wastes from the cell. Sodium and potassium ratios are extremely important to this flow. Potassium within the cell wall opposes the absorption of salts. If the body lacks this nutrient, salt will enter the cells and draw water into the cell. We call this "holding fluid" and can be demonstrated by a finger poke to a puffy part of the skin. It will turn white if holding fluid. Leg cramps may also indicate low of potassium.

Follow Others: Aging Wisdom from Beatitudes, Nature, Kinfolk

Holding Fluids on a Cruise. My daughter-in-law noticed extreme swelling of her ankles when onboard a cruise ship. Research uncovered that drinking water on board is obtained through water desalination and may have traces of salt. They plan to bring canned water on their next cruise.

Ways to prevent holding fluid:

Limit salt intake; read labels on prepared foods; look for low-salt versions. Read Salt Sensitivity in Chapter 8.

Increase consumption of protein.

Bananas, potatoes, leafy greens and chocolate are good sources of potassium.

Shaklee's Alfalfa tabs are a clean source of potassium.

Copper and Zinc Facts. The body requires that trace minerals such as copper and zinc be taken in balance. Enough zinc in our diets in this day of copper plumbing is difficult, as tap water will always contain some copper.

Issues about zinc are given below:

Zinc is important to skin health. Baby ointments contain zinc and vitamin D and have been slathered on baby bottoms for decades.

Zinc helps ward off colds; there is a homeopathic remedy that contains zinc and is sold for that purpose. Protects against Covid19 cell replication.

A healthy prostate gland needs zinc, which is found in male ejaculate.

Sources of Zinc: Fresh fruits; Zinc supplements are available in 10 mg and 50 mg (typical) tablets.

Follow Others: Aging Wisdom from Beatitudes, Nature, Kinfolk

Oily vs. Water-soluble Vitamins – Facts. Have you heard warnings on TV, the internet, newspapers or magazines to beware of vitamins? These warnings are only partially true. The fact not mentioned is that there is a large difference in how our bodies utilize oily vs. water-soluble vitamins.

Oily vitamins such as vitamin A, D and E can remain in the body IF taken in very large doses and frequently. This could cause damage, but can be entirely prevented by smaller doses taken less frequently and in balance with other vitamins (hence the popularity of multivitamin tablets). Since A & D are oily vitamins, you can take larger amounts in the winter when oil is sluggish. In warmer weather, you should reduce the amount of oily vitamin A, especially.

Water-soluble vitamins, such as all the B-vitamins and C, need to be renewed daily in order to keep our bodies healthy. These wash out in the urine and are extremely safe. Even if taken in high-dosages, one only needs to stop and they will all come out "in the wash" so to speak. And don't let doctors scare you about the money wasted on large doses that simply color your urine. I once listened to my doctor and cut down my larger dose of Vitamin C. Within weeks I spotted the first wrinkle on my face—a line between my eyebrows. It has never gone away.

End Point: Read chapter 8 for Generic Aging recommendations.

Prayer Point: Beatitude according to Luke—But woe unto you that are rich! for ye have received your consolation. Luke 6:24

Follow Others: Aging Wisdom from Beatitudes, Nature, Kinfolk
Part 3: Exercise

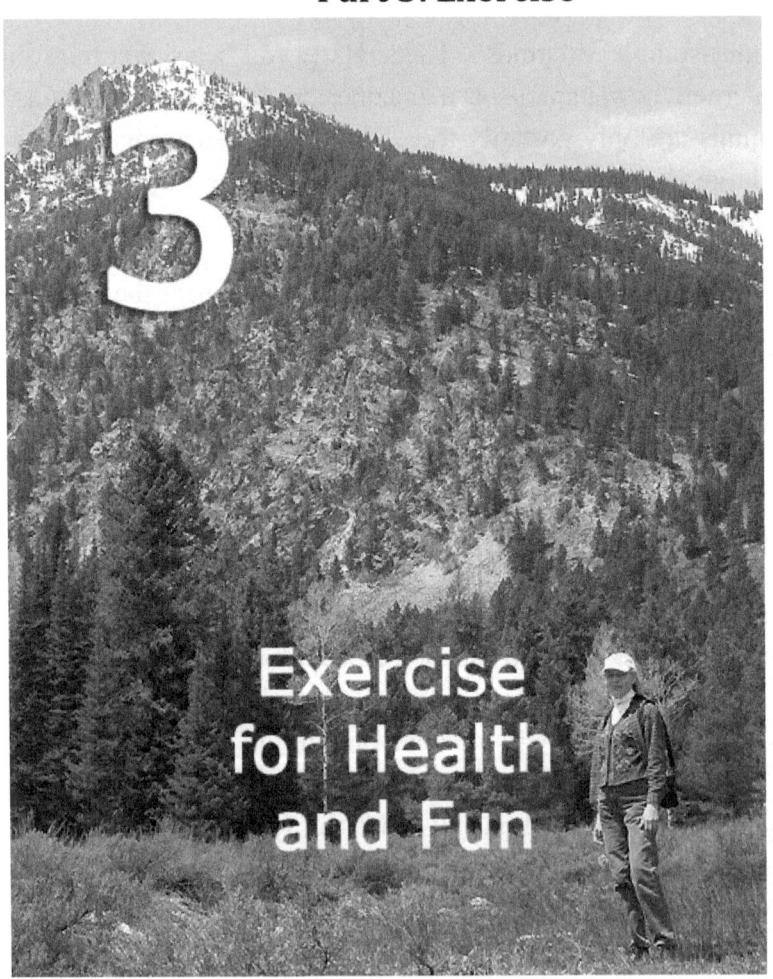

In This Part...

Chap10: Adventure Stirs the Bones

Chap11: Diet Fads and Fitness

Chap12: Motivation in Motion

Follow Others: Aging Wisdom from Beatitudes, Nature, Kinfolk

Beatitude: Blessed and happy and enviably fortunate, and spiritually prosperous [that is, with life-joy and satisfaction in God's favor and salvation, regardless of your outward conditions]—are you when people revile you and persecute you and say all kinds of evil things against your falsely on My account, Be gland and supremely joyful, for your reward in heaven is great (strong and intense), for in this same way people persecuted the prophets who were before you. Matthew 5:11-12 Amplified

Chapter 10—Adventure Stirs the Bones

Once I got over the forced retirement by my company, I decided to find a hobby. It had to be something that I always wished to do. Having read the book Drawing on the Right Side of the Brain, I considered painting as a retirement hobby. I even purchased a lot of brushes and an easel with books on how to use oils and watercolors in anticipation. I knew a former co-worker who did just that. Both Winston Churchill and Grandma Moses are well-known as retiree painters.

Reading Betty Edwards book on drawing/painting will put you in touch with your creative side (right brain) which is especially helpful to those who are analytical (left brain) like myself. Guess what? Painting no longer stirs my bones. My hand-eye coordination is lacking, for one reason. As a writer, I already spend too much time sitting. Look at some of the opportunities I have been pursuing instead.

Mineral and Gold Hunt – Author

I remembered my fascination with rocks that began in third grade. The Hartford housing project where we lived was still under development. There were chunks of quartz and mica, fill stone everywhere. All I had to do was look down to find a sparkly "treasure" to place in my bureau drawer.

Follow Others: Aging Wisdom from Beatitudes, Nature, Kinfolk

One day I stayed home from school due to nausea. When I opened that drawer, the rocks inside looked brown and lack luster and made me feel literally ill. I threw them all away.

After retirement, the idea to study stones and minerals excited me. (After all, I had relatives on both sides who worked with stones; Read their stories in this book.) I bought tiny samples stuck to a board and books with full-color pictures. Our New Hampshire back yard offered me plenty of opportunities to apply what I was learning. Once again, I put hand-picked samples in a box or on a shelf.

Our gold panning and rock hunting adventures netted us little except experience. And exercise, because whatever stirs our bones, gets us up and moving. You'll never guess what I almost did this weekend? At a nearby mineral club show, I looked into taking a geology course at a local University. Go Adventure!

About the Photo: The picture at the start of Part 3 was taken in 2003. The author in her sixties was on a lower mountain trail in Wyoming. In 2018 she climbed a 1.1 mile trail up a New Hampshire mountain peak that was 800 ft. high.

Cook and Baker Skills – Author

Of English heritage, I love tea and baked goods associated with Victorian tea parties. In case I decided to open my own tea room, I took a college course in baking. I learned all about the chemistry of baking ingredients and gained hands-on skills in the creation of pastries to delight any Englishwoman.

The tea room never materialized, although I have some graceful tea services with cups and saucers that sit behind glass doors, waiting to make a debut when my next book goes to print.

Follow Others: Aging Wisdom from Beatitudes, Nature, Kinfolk

Tea Choices. My father-in-law once said that you didn't have to buy fancy teas; you could simply brew up the lawn clippings. He preferred coffee, of course; though it was his wife who taught me to enjoy a tea party. I own some pieces from her lovely tea service nowadays.

Suggestions for choosing the right tea. Teas are medicinal since they derive from herbs and fruits with healing or invigorating properties. If you have tried one type of tea and made the decision that you don't like them, it was probably because you tried the wrong tea. I always suggest to people who are leery of tea that they try a sip or two of a new tea flavor someone offers them. Be brave and you may just find a healthy "friend" for life.

Green tea (decaf or regular) is recommended for everyone's health. I drink this at breakfast.

Herbal teas target particular health issues. Peppermint tea calms an upset tummy. Chamomile soothes teething pain and fights against colds.

There is a tea to suit everyone's body chemistry. For example, people who have a strong thyroid gland will actually lose weight if they drink raspberry tea. Others who have a strong adrenal gland will find parsley tea consumed at lunch time cuts down their mid-afternoon hunger for salt, nuts and cheese. For information on diet by body type, read chapter 11.

Food Tailored to Health Issues. Once I realized that I have a salt sensitivity which elevates my blood pressure, I began the search for prepared foods that are low salt and seasoned with herbs. Good luck trying. Either these foods are totally bland (you can at least add herbs to those) or so salty they don't even taste good.

Follow Others: Aging Wisdom from Beatitudes, Nature, Kinfolk

Home delivery systems. I joined HelloFresh and have stayed with them for several reasons. Other systems deliver prepared foods to your home with labels indicating specialties such as Gluten-Free and Salt Sensitive. You may find a local kitchen that does.

Here are the reasons why I stay with HelloFresh:

I learn new cooking skills. I had never made risotto before. And never tried any Asian spice recipes.

I can control how much salt I add by substituting herbs whenever salt is called for or I can substitute unsalted butter and broths.

With the need to preorder meals, there is now more variety in our diet, instead of the constant replay of ten favorite recipes.

These often present a Mediterranean/Asian food plan with many healthy food choices. FYI, the Mediterranean diet is currently considered the most healthy diet there is. Read Chapter 11.

Pickup or Delivery. Target, Walmart and Stop & Shop stores now allow you to order online with delivery options. I don't have to go to the store and shop so frequently.

Travel as Education. Many retirees take vacations that introduce them to parts of the world they might not otherwise visit. Church groups sponsor trips to the Holy Land. You can take cruises to Alaska, the Caribbean, Scandinavia and Europe.

Before taking a trip by air, land or sea consider suggestions on making sure your body enjoys the adventure. For example:

Digestive Issues - See other tips in section at the end of this chapter.

Follow Others: Aging Wisdom from Beatitudes, Nature, Kinfolk

Motion sickness help: Wear a band at the wrist that activates pressure points; On a cruise, get a cabin located mid-ships; Bring Dramamine or take B-6.

Water consumption: Purify any water drunk on camping trips; Do not drink water while travelling out of the country; Holding fluid on Cruises is discussed in Chapter 9.

Find Your Adventure

Club Memberships. Early American settlers were accused of being less well-educated than their British counterparts. So people throughout the early states participated in Clubs to continue learning. Ralph Waldo Emerson is well known for his Transcendental Club near Boston; Abraham Lincoln also joined a reading club on the edge of what was then the wilderness.

As we age, we can continue to learn by joining clubs. Whether we go on hikes or meet at Barnes & Noble for their monthly book club, doing so can keep us mentally spry or physically spunky. Spry and spunky sound full of adventure, right?

Maybe you'll find some challenge listed below. Or add a new adventure that speaks to you, then set a goal and get started.

Travel

Outdoors – hike, fish, hunt gold and gems

Marathons

Volunteer

Politics

Hobby – paint, rock hunting

Follow Others: Aging Wisdom from Beatitudes, Nature, Kinfolk

Cooking Class

Video/archive for family

Restore Vehicle

Write book – memoir, novel

Coin Collecting

Collecting National and International Coins. A co-worker started collecting coins when he was about 10 with an order to Littleton Company, from an ad in a magazine. You may not realize that this hobby's fascination is due to the international nature of the hobby. In his own words:

"Most of the youngsters, boys most of them, started collecting coins or stamps that way at the time. They sent you packets monthly of coins on approval, and if you had a little bit of newspaper delivery money to spend, you could purchase them that way.

A few years later I found a local coin shop, where you can browse through the glass display cases and learn and dream about how coins relate to each other, or what far-away countries they were from. I saw my first ancient Roman coin at a shop like this, a bronze coin from the time of Constantine the Great. I never forgot holding something almost two thousand years in my hand.

This collecting hobby is not too expensive for seniors, with coins you can collect from all over the world for pennies, or even find in pocket change. The biggest problem I have collecting is my eyes. You need a very good lighted magnifier to see much by way of dates or mint marks."

But that's not enough to stop my coworker from collecting.

Follow Others: Aging Wisdom from Beatitudes, Nature, Kinfolk

Be Active

Runners–My third son ran his first race in 2018 at the age of forty-eight. He has been an elected member of local boards, including Zoning board.

Don't Follow the Old Man. Here's a funny, true story about older runners told by the preacher, Jesse Duplantis. This Cajun preacher tells of a marathon he ran up and down a mountainous road on an Hawaiian island. He followed a runner who was much older. That runner told him not to give up, which infuriated Duplantis' pride. He wouldn't quit keeping up even with painful swollen knees on the downhill run. When Duplantis complained to the Lord, he was told to "quit following the 92-year-old man." Pride can suck all the joy out of exercise and adventures, with conscquences that may take a long time to heal.

I recently read in The Longevity Paradox that running long-distance races can cause scarring of the right ventricular heart muscle. Everything in moderation.

Politics, Another Way to Run – Sarah Palin. Prior to her national recognition, Palin ran for local offices including Mayor of her town. Sarah "still felt a restlessness, and insistent tugging on her heart"… [t]hat there were other ways she could contribute. "So I ran for governor" of the state, Alaska. With limited budget, the campaign trail for the Governor's election put her in her car throughout a long snowy winter of dark days. To attend meet and great events around the state, she once crossed Thompson Pass driving in snow with her small children asleep in the backseat of her VW Jetta.

Follow Others: Aging Wisdom from Beatitudes, Nature, Kinfolk

Unlike many other candidates who promise change, Palin delivered after each win. Those she defeated never expected to be unseated. Nor did they expect that she would 'clean house' of hangers-on who refused to cooperate with her promised goals. As she described that determination in her biography, "You can't blink... You have to be wired in a way of being so committed to the mission." She wasn't called "Sarah Barracuda" by her high school basketball team mates for nothing!

Her Heritage/Legacy. Sarah Palin was raised to believe that everyone can make a difference. This is understandable since she is related through her parents to five Pilgrim families that arrived in Plymouth on the Mayflower in 1620. Her father, Charles (Chuck) Heath, is related to Henry Samson. Her mother, Sarah (Sally) Sheeran, is descended from heads of four Mayflower families: John Howland, Richard Warren, Giles and Stephen Hopkins and William Brewster (religious leader and advisor to Plymouth colony's governor).

With her father a science teacher and school coach, Sarah's interest in nature and sports is hardly surprising. Posted on Facebook : her "favorite movies are sports related..."it's all about the underdog, the unconventional, the character revealed in over comers." From her own sports experience, Sarah "knew the guts it takes to run." She also played high school basketball; with her help their team won the 1982 Alaska state championship.

Since childhood Sarah was interested in government and current events. As a teen she remembers President Ronald Reagan's common sense public policy. In college, she was intrigued by political science classes and she chose journalism as her major—she realized that "words held power."

(Extracted sections from the author's book, Miracle of the Call.)

Follow Others: Aging Wisdom from Beatitudes, Nature, Kinfolk

A Legacy of Volunteering. I loved volunteering when my children were young and I stayed at home to be with them. I collected good, used clothing to give away for free in a small shop over our church meeting hall. I didn't realize that my efforts were doubly rewarded. My service provided free clothing for my four fast-growing children—a second job without the need to leave home. Towns people came for clothes and I invited them and their children to our church activities. One of these younger women became my sister-in-law.

Below are stories of how my service has passed along to my four children. Three sons all have had their pictures in their local Northeast newspaper or on television. My daughter will see her recognition for church service once she reaches heaven.

Volunteer Emergency Response. Chuck, my oldest son has volunteered for the Red Cross and now as an associate sheriff in the Springfield, MA, area. He has often been on TV as spokesperson for fires and weather events.

Volunteer fire fighter. Matthew F

Stafford Zoning Commission board. Dan F

Volunteer office staff for Christian radio station and churches. Grace T

Volunteer at a local soup kitchen once a month for two years. Walt and Grace T

Follow Others: Aging Wisdom from Beatitudes, Nature, Kinfolk

Don't Let Digestive Issues Stop Adventure. Some people never launch an adventure or travel far from home simply because their alimentary canal functions can't handle different water and different foods, such as lots of beans and rice. Anyone else's hand in the air along with mine?

Indigestion Solutions. Here are some facts that your parents or teachers never mentioned. And probably not your doctor either. Discomfort may result also from yo-yo dieting.

Lactaid. Milk products, such as butter, cheese and yogurt, are used in many cuisines. Make sure you take Lactaid tablets in sealed packets with you. Chew one or more tablets, if you suspect dairy is used in a meal; definitely if you eat lots of ice cream over summer travels.

Probiotics. Probiotics maintain normal gut level balance of good versus bad microscopic creatures that are normally found in the intestines. Take regularly before, during and after travel. There are many kinds that need no refrigeration

Food Poisoning. There are several good remedies useful against food poisoning. Most are portable or readily available. Homeopathic remedies – Nux Vomica and Arsenicum Albanus, both available in tubes of 30C sugar pills. Nux Vomica can be used to settle stomach rumbles no matter which category they arrive in. Arsenicum Albanus is for food poisoning, such as eating out-dated or under-heated leftovers.

Gall Bladder Issues. You may have experienced gall bladder pain under your right ribs, or have had your gall bladder removed. Lemons are the only food that is a substitute for bile in the digestive process. Cut one lemon lengthwise into 4 or 6 slices. Suck a slice or squeeze and drink the lemon juice after a greasy meal or one with lots of fat like mayonnaise.

Follow Others: Aging Wisdom from Beatitudes, Nature, Kinfolk

International Bugs/Parasites. Rule number 1: Don't eat or drink ANYTHING that has not been boiled/cooked. Rule number 2: Get all of the shots recommended for the area to which you will be going. You may be against the concept of vaccination, but if you get a disease, you'll wish the rest of your life you had listened.

Elimination Fixes

Role of Water Supply. The calcium/magnesium found in any given water supply can have negative effects if different than what your body is used to. You may experience constipation, diarrhea or kidney stones.

For stateside travel, drink ONLY bottled water. This includes hot drinks such as water or tea. Since restaurants use local water for their hot drinks, you'll have to take your chances. At least any negative consequences (diarrhea) will not be long-lasting.

For overseas travel, NEVER drink local water or eat raw produce. There could be parasites.

Hard stuff – Constipation. There are many portable options to overcome this stubborn bowel problem.

Bring your regular laxative with you. Plan on taking a smaller, less frequent doses because diarrhea may occur after drinking water from other sources

Bring fiber gummies, but don't take too many. Sorbitol and other artificial sweeteners have a mild laxative effect.

Miralax is a stool softener you may already have taken after a surgery.

Follow Others: Aging Wisdom from Beatitudes, Nature, Kinfolk

Soft stuff – Diarrhea. There are fewer options to overcome this bowel issue which can result from foods not normally consumed. The last one in this list of portable remedies will be a surprise:

Homeopathic – Nux Vomica, available in tubes of 30C sugar pills

OTC remedies, such as Imodium; wait until stomach is empty

Carob powder – Only use this remedy if diarrhea is long-standing and accompanied by vomiting. See my cautionary Carob story below. Seems funnier when it's someone else's story.

Carob for Diarrhea – My Funny Story. My spouse had an ongoing bout with diarrhea. OTC remedies were not working. On a visit to our local health food/vitamin shop, I asked the owner what she would recommend. She told me to mix one heaped TBSP of Carob powder into a small amount of heated water in a cup—kind like hot chocolate without milk. I gave it to my spouse, and his diarrhea stopped completely. Who would think?

Shortly afterwards, I caught the bug and started with the same negative effects, except that I seldom vomit. So I was still eating small amounts of food, and my intestinal tract was not empty.

Impressed with the results carob had for my spouse, I mixed the hot drink for myself. I did not count on what would happen if food was still in my system. As I groaned with intestinal discomfort that night, nothing moved in either direction for awhile. I had to laugh at how foolish I had been to take advice from an unknown woman in a health food store. Though I still keep Carob powder for just such an emergency.

CAUTION: Don't take carob powder to stop diarrhea if you are still eating food. Like OTC Imodium, wait until your stomach is empty.

Follow Others: Aging Wisdom from Beatitudes, Nature, Kinfolk

Probiotics, Prebiotics and Cultured Foods. The Russian biologist, Elie Metchnikoff, who first advocated for probiotics in 1910 had discovered the connection between aging and poor gut health. This Nobel Prize recipient was not believed at first, but nowadays nearly everyone prescribed an antibiotic knows that yogurt can reduce the number of good bacteria killed in the bowel.

FYI, prebiotics are good sources for probiotics. I will use the term probiotics because that was how the 1970s addressed them.

Who Needs Probiotics? Those on antibiotics? Yes, however, everyone needs these foods that feed your healthy probiotics colony. And that is why if you search the internet for cultured foods, such as yogurt, you will discover that every culture has a fermented favorite, such as kimchi, included in their diet.

What happens when you take probiotics? Good, Bad and not so Ugly.

Good – Normal Intestinal Environment. A daily probiotics capsule, along with changed eating habits, can help return a normal intestinal environment. This will:

Decrease intestinal permeability, and therefore decrease food sensitivity.

Increase production of B vitamins, A and K as per a healthy bowel.

Increase absorption of minerals from your food.

Read The Longevity Paradox for the newest information.

Follow Others: Aging Wisdom from Beatitudes, Nature, Kinfolk

Bad – Yeast Infection. Candidiasis is a fungal disease which can take over bacterial colonies in mucous-lined tissues such as found in the mouth, vagina and intestine. It is normally found in the body. However, taking antibiotics allow this yeast to thrive in the intestine and change into a fungus which can slip through weakened intestinal walls. It can then travel through the body, including the brain, to cause immune system issues such as food allergies.

Probiotics are advised along with a lengthy (6 month) abstinence from yeast-feeding foods such as bread and carbohydrates.

Not So Ugly – Cultured Foods Around the World. What do yogurt and kimchi have in common? These are both native foods that forestall/prevent the intestinal overgrowth by bacteria that cause fungal disease. No need to pack yogurt if you head out to a global country, but you might prefer to take a few probiotics pills along rather than smell like fermented cabbage (kimchi)*.

*American troops stationed in Korea after the war, did not permit their paid houseboys to make kimchi in the barracks because of the smell. Nowadays, it is a popular spicy condiment.

End Point: "It is God to whom and with whom we travel, and while He is the end of our journey, He is also at every stopping place." Elisabeth Elliot

Prayer Point: Beatitude according to Luke—Woe unto you that are full! for ye shall hunger. Luke 6:25a

Follow Others: Aging Wisdom from Beatitudes, Nature, Kinfolk

Beatitude: You are the salt of the earth, but if the salt has lost its taste—its strength, its quality—how can its saltiness be restored? It is not good for anything any longer but to be thrown out and trodden under foot by men. 5:13 Amplified

Chapter 11—Diet Fads and Fitness

Exercise and Diet Plans are strategies seniors can employ to stay healthy and alive. Choosing the best plan(s) for your body type etc. is so important, that this chapter will explain in some depth options relatively unknown and whether or not these are healthy. After all, eating only grapefruit or all meat diets makes no sense, no matter how desperately we want to believe in them.

What makes those of us with Blood Type A act like a bunch of hypochondriacs, you ask? Others around us are seldom sickly. Their colds disappear quickly, but we get bronchitis instead. After a while you just want to do something—anything proactive—so that people will stop asking why you are sick again. One benefit is that I learned a great deal about nutrition and supplementation. Read chapters 6-9, especially, to see the knowledge I've shared in this book about nutrition and health.

New research on aging concludes, that people who stay thin or lose weight do not age as quickly as those who don't. This is because the more food we consume, the more chances that free radicals will occur and disrupt the health of our DNA. That's a pretty good lead-in to the topics of diet and exercise.

Follow Others: Aging Wisdom from Beatitudes, Nature, Kinfolk

Diet Myths. People make wrong assumptions about diets (and vitamin supplements, too, for that matter).

One diet plan should fit all—For decades proponents of low-carb diets have argued with those who swear by high-fat diets. If one diet were ideal, by now it would have proved successful for all body types. None has. Read the next two sections on Blood Type and Body Type diets to get help in finding the perfect combination of diet and foods to eat which work specifically for you.

A diet is a crutch—What it does is free you for the time being from eating your addictive foods, which like a drug can trigger an inappropriate hunger response.

A diet is something only need to follow once—like wonder-working antibiotics. Such faulty assumptions include: Start a diet today, lose the weight and expect it will never come back. Equally foolish is to take a calcium tablet for a month and expect your leg muscles will never cramp again.

If you fall off a diet you may as well quit—The truth is that everyone eats things they should not while on a diet. Here is the advice I've personally used for years. If you eat something wrong, you still have to eat the right thing, too. After getting uncomfortably stuffed a few times, you will not so quickly fall off the diet.

Fasting for Fat Burning. Interest in dietary fasting has resurfaced due to Keto diet plans. Here are some truths about the confusing information on fasting. To burn or not to burn fat:

A one day fast is only a body-cleansing fast; it does not burn fat.

Fasts that last 3 days or longer do burn fat. You will recognize when your body goes into ketosis by these changes: tongue changes color; bad taste in mouth; Low energy or extremely tired

Follow Others: Aging Wisdom from Beatitudes, Nature, Kinfolk

Taking a ketone supplement to provoke fat burning is less healthy over the long term.

Other Fasting Facts. Fasts of various types will cleanse the body but may or may not burn fat:

Liquid fast – broth and juices with water (pre-surgery type fast)

Water alone with a bit of lemon juice**

First meal after a fast should be a salad or other light but nutritious foods.

IMPORTANT: People who are hypoglycemic or diabetic should not opt for a water or water and lemon only fast. They may experience light-headedness or fainting. Add in liquid-like applesauce or yogurt.

Customized Health and Diet Plans. My Orthopedic doctor once told me, that I controlled my genetic weaknesses by diet. And, yes, you too can create a customized diet using plans in this section.

"A diet is a program of change in the areas of behavior and attitudes about food and exercise." Jonny Bowden. In the Greek the word means a manner of living. To make it easier to evaluate them, I provide a rather detailed analysis of each diet. For specific information, recipes and/or meal plans, purchase the books mentioned in the Resources at end of this book.

Several diet plans mentioned in this section are customized for your individual body type. These plans provide specific information about the foods and eating styles that best suit you: Eating for blood type; Eating for strongest gland. Other diet plans mentioned are more generic and will work for anyone who chooses and sticks to the plan that is best

Follow Others: Aging Wisdom from Beatitudes, Nature, Kinfolk

for them. Many diet plans advertised on TV currently offer testing in order to customize for your body or bloody type. One now uses DNA testing.

"The tongue of the wise is health." Proverbs 12:18

Blood Type – What does it have to do with diet?

Do you know anyone who has been sickly all of their lives? Or maybe this describes you? Your blood type may be at fault—definitely so if you have blood type A, either positive or negative. Give me a few minutes to set the stage and I'll discuss that troublesome blood type A.

We inherit our blood type from one of our parents. My father was a blood type O and my mother a blood type A. With only two choices, I ended up type A. I have five siblings who may be either A or O blood type due to genetics. I will tell you that blood type A and O are the most prevalent in the Western world. Scientists believe blood type A comes from Western Europe. And the other blood types developed as tribes moved to Eastern Europe.

About that pesky blood type A! My mother was sickly from her teens onward. Her relatives tried to get her to eat liverwurst sandwiches for lunch to help build up her blood. I was her first born and the only child she nursed. She worried that I was constipated as an infant and immediately started me on laxatives. All my siblings got enemas as the magic cure for any illness in the family. In her defense, blood type As are more prone to anxiety than type O.

When in my 20s, I remember that my health and then that of my children caused me the most concern. (My husband worried about the car.) Opposite of my mother, I was more interested in the food I consumed, and researched vitamins, herbs and then homeopathic remedies as answers to ward off illness.

Follow Others: Aging Wisdom from Beatitudes, Nature, Kinfolk

About Blood Types – Eat Right 4 Your Type. At a friend's home seven years ago I came across this book by Dr. Peter J. D'Adamo. Finally, I had my answer to hypochondria, blood type-A style. Guess what? It gets worse! Type A people are inclined toward having Leukemia and dying early of heart issues. Now there really was something to be concerned about. Fortunately, I had embarked on healthy eating styles early on, and already related the food I ate with resistance to disease. Also, I've spent oodles of time and money on food supplements.

Meal Planning by Blood Type. D'Adamo's book contains a complete list of all dairy, grains, vegetables, fruit, meats and seafood, oils and even spices. Follow the column for your blood type to see whether you should avoid a food, consider it neutral or recognize that it is beneficial to your body. What a marvelous tool!

Interestingly enough, your body already has agreed with most of these findings. My ex-husband and current spouse both have blood type O. They can eat meat without harmful side effects; they actually thrive on it. I do enjoy an occasional steak, but fish, turkey and chicken are my favorite protein choices. No wonder my mom gave away those liverwurst sandwiches made by her aunt for her! Or that I always preferred fish to meats, liked beets and avocado and more recently disliked fructose-type sugars.

Not a Diet Plan – What happens when you eat for blood type?. You may or may not lose weight, but this method of eating can help prevent unhealthy food interactions in the body. Depending on blood type, D'Adamo's book warns that certain foods cause cell bindings that can harm an individual. Unhealthy cell bindings may contribute to autoimmune responses, brown spots on the skin and leaky gut syndrome.

Follow Others: Aging Wisdom from Beatitudes, Nature, Kinfolk

Unhealthy bindings: Agglutinins – bind with antibodies; Lectins – proteins in outer skins/seed that can cause cells to bind; Indican levels – raised levels are associated with bacterial activity in the intestines causing poor digestion and leaky gut

Body Type Diet. My ex-husband was vacuuming the house on his day off (nice guy), and learned about this diet on TV. When I got home, he told me that it would be perfect for me. I had been gaining weight impossible to shed ever since I started my sit-down job as a technical writer. Results came once I applied the book's information, shifted a few foods around and limited others. I have never weighed over 135 pounds while adhering to that diet.

About Strongest Glands. Dr Abravanel's Body Type Diet and Lifetime Nutrition Plan book begins with the premise that each of us has one stronger endocrine gland and we learn to rely on that gland for energy. Energy is generated when we eat and digest (trigger) foods specific to that gland. Unfortunately, decades later our body tires out the strongest gland simply because we can't stop eating these foods. And more embarrassingly, we gain all our weight in specific places, often labeled beer belly or love handles.

Here is a list of the glands and trigger foods discussed in his book:

Thyroid: Trigger foods: Caffeine and Carbs—Fat location: love handles, biceps

Adrenal: Trigger foods: Salt, Fat, Red Meat, Alcohol, Nuts, Eggs—Fat location: Belly and kidney area

Pituitary: Trigger foods: Dairy products—Fat location: All over the body—puffy hands etc.

Gonad: Trigger foods: Spicy foods—Fat location: Hip area

Follow Others: Aging Wisdom from Beatitudes, Nature, Kinfolk

Quiz, Meal Plans and Timing. Follow these steps to lose weight and keep it off:

Take the quiz provided in the book to learn which is your strongest gland.

Use information from the book to determine the best time for your meals. For those who I call Thyroid people, plan to eat your biggest meal at lunch. For Adrenal people, plan to eat light until evening.

Limit what foods you eat in the morning so your most-tired gland can have time to recover. Always eat trigger foods for other glands at breakfast. Eggs for Thyroid people, are an excellent choice. Adrenal people, like myself, need a cup of tea or coffee with caffeine in order to be creative that day. Save your gland's trigger foods for evening. For example, since my adrenal gland is the strongest, I should never eat eggs for breakfast, otherwise I will be hungry all day. If a Thyroid person has some carbs, like cereals for a supper meal, there isn't enough left of the day to overindulge with more sweets.

After following the basic weight loss plan for a length of time and stuck at a plateau, switch to the appropriate type soup diet for a week or less to burn cellulite and then back-to-basic diet. Occasionally, check to see that you haven't wandered off of the maintenance diet, especially if your scale reports a weight increase.

More Diet Plans – Health at the Table. Choose a generic type among this assortment of long-time diet plans as well as several newest ones.

Count Calories. If you eat more calories than you burn, you will gain weight. There are many fancier diet types, but plans that track/limit calories are still successful strategies for weight loss and maintenance.

Follow Others: Aging Wisdom from Beatitudes, Nature, Kinfolk

Recommended calories for adult male and females, based on age and life style:

Female – young—Sedentary: 1,800; Active: 2,400

Female – over 50—Sedentary: 1,600; Active: 2,000

Male – young—Sedentary: 2,600; Active: 2,800

Male – over 70—Sedentary: 2,000; Active: 2,600

Daily calorie totals should be divided between three meals. You may consider a meal replacement per day or supplemental vitamin and protein mix to make sure you get the correct number of calories as you diet. See the internet for more information and sample diet plans.

Weigh-In and Accountability. Weight Watchers uses the counting calories methodology, but reinforces it with goals, weekly weigh-ins, DNA testing and fees. Many workplaces use similar strategies to keep their employees up-and-moving and healthy. Some provide employees with fit-bits or other wrist indicators that count steps.

Meal Replacement and Supplemental Programs. Companies that produce nutritional supplements also sell Protein drinks. Some of these products are supplements to support a diet and exercise plan, while other mixes are meant to replace one or more meals per day. Check the product information and labels to make sure you purchase the right protein product.

High/Low Fat. Diets have been around for several decades that recommend you consume high fats and even low-fat foods. There has been much debate about which works best to help you lose weight.

Follow Others: Aging Wisdom from Beatitudes, Nature, Kinfolk

Refer to the Body Type Diet section to learn whether consumption of high or low-fat foods might be best for you. Sample diets for each type of these diets can be found in book stores and online.

Newest Diets—The major goal of the newest diets is weight reduction by fat-burning, improved health and/or healthy eating habits.

Anti-Inflammatory. The AI diet recommends a healthy balance of nutrient-dense foods that include proteins, carbohydrates, and fats plus fruits. It differs from a standard diet in the removal of foods that trigger inflammation for a six-month period. This diet can treat obesity, arthritis and irritable bowel syndrome. Sample diet plans and recipes can be found in book stores and online.

Paleo. This diet limits the types of foods included in their meal plans to only the foods that were available to early mankind. This excludes cooked grains. Since cooked grains are high in calories, this diet will work similarly as counting calories. And it does guarantee you will eat lots of healthy meats and raw fruits and vegetables. Sample diet plans and recipes can be found in book stores and online.

Keto. These diets encourage the rapid burning of stored body fat. They promote high-fat, low-to-moderate protein and low-carb foods with taking ketone supplements. This diet will work similarly to a high-fat diet. The difference is that the goal is to put your body quickly into a ketosis state to guarantee rapid fat burning. This will help burn stubborn cellulite and move past your current weight loss plateau. It will also allow the body to detox from sugar. See the Body Type Diet for other methods to move past plateaus and burn cellulite.

CAUTION: To prevent damage to healthy tissues in the body, ketosis (definition below) initiated by diet plans should be limited to short durations of several days or a week. Starvation can set in at the cell level when fat supplies are exhausted; then the body will burn protein.

Ketosis Defined. When a person's regular food supply is withdrawn, such as a fast or times of famine, the body begins to burn its stored fat. This puts the body in ketosis. A low-grade fuel, such as stored fat, burns so that the body develops a bad taste in the mouth, has less energy and acts tired. In the past when I tried a fast, I felt too tired to do much except rest, read or meditate. Perhaps that's why people have fasted in the past for religious reasons.

Read a previous section on Fasting Myths.

Health-Specific Diets – Most diets have weight-loss as a motive. As we age, however, more diets have health concerns as the chief motivation. This is a quick overview of some health-specific diets. Doctors will provide plans for you to follow, many are similar to popular weight-loss diets. This is because the body suffers from overweight and/or low-weight conditions.

High/Low Blood Sugar. Civilized people's eat large amounts of sugar—maybe as much as a pound in a year. Fruits contain sugar but fiber and water as well. Dried fruit and baked sweets allow a person to eat huge amounts of sugar that can damage the pancreas.

High blood sugar – can damage the pancreas which is the source of insulin.

Low blood sugar – Rapid drop over one hour period causes many symptoms of low blood sugar, such as a foggy mind, feelings of starvation and anti-social behavior. Beta blockers taken for high blood pressure can intensify low blood sugar spikes/drops; take smaller amounts twice a day.

Follow Others: Aging Wisdom from Beatitudes, Nature, Kinfolk

Glucose Tolerance Testing. Fasting blood sugar levels should be under 90; 120 is a typical blood sugar level after eating. The test requires the candidate to drink a highly-sweetened drink; blood is drawn at intervals from 1-3 hours or 1- 5 hours. Plotting a chart of these levels against time gives a picture of whether the person has high, low or normal blood sugar and also at what rate it rises and drops.

Diabetic/Pre-diabetes Diet Plans. These diets replace sugar in the diet with artificial sweetened foods. Many of these artificial sweeteners can cause stomach and bowel issues. They award points to various types of foods, so the diabetic need not count calories.

Tips for artificial sweeteners: Stevia, a naturally sweet leaf, is the current favorite. Monkfruit is another current favorite; Limit sugar alcohols like mannitol which can cause diarrhea; Limit manufactured sugar substitutes, like Splenda. These can cause kidney issues; Aspartame can cause autoimmune symptoms, like Lupus or Fibromyalgia.

Refer to the diet plan provided by your doctor or nutritionist. Chromium tablets can reduce the cravings for sweet foods.

Diabetes – Late Onset – Consult a doctor immediately. Do you crave sugar or at least tolerate it now, when you did not earlier in life? This can indicate late-onset Diabetes. My father had it, my mother-in-law and my spouse's mother. Patients who are near death in a nursing home want only ice cream (loaded with sugar).

Here are some explanations why we crave sugar when we are aging:

Our pancreas is no longer able to produce the full amount of insulin. Cells cannot receive/use the nutrition from food to generate energy needed for health. Food we eat contains two of the known eight sugars. Six must be manufactured by healthy cells. Our cells know that if they

Follow Others: Aging Wisdom from Beatitudes, Nature, Kinfolk

get more sugar they should be able to create the needed energy. This is true in a healthy body within a toxic-free environment. Unfortunately, those with serious illnesses like Louis Gehrig's disease and cancer, have bodies that are toxic. Even beached whales suffer from a toxic environment.

The six sugars manufactured in the body support specific organ health. One of these six is responsible for breast health. Other endocrine glands may be tired out from eating too many trigger foods. See Dr. Abranavel diet. Refer to website for www.Mannatech.com for more information on Mannatech's Ambrotose complex which contains all eight sugars.

Specific test methods are: glucose meter to track daily A1C level (should remain in range of 5 to 6 for a diabetic); routine lab work. Meal planning is an important tool for maintenance of the A1C target.

Feet – Signs in doctor offices request diabetes patients to remove shoes for physicals. Diabetes can cause nerve damage in the feet.

Kidney – Holding urine can harm the small blood vessels in the kidney. Urine and blood tests can pinpoint any problems before they become a health risk.

Eyes – Small blood vessels in the eyes can also be damaged by high blood sugar.

Cholesterol Prevention Diet. Your liver (see section below) makes most of the cholesterol your body needs to build cells. This waxy substance can build up in arteries (atherosclerosis) and cause blockages. The rest of your cholesterol comes from animal food products. It is the combination of low HDL and high LDL that can cause heart attacks.

Good vs. Bad Cholesterol. HDL (good) cholesterol needs levels of 40 (men), 50 (women) to 60 mg/dL in order to prevent heart attacks from high LDL. If HDL is too low, a doctor may recommend the B-vitamin

Follow Others: Aging Wisdom from Beatitudes, Nature, Kinfolk

Niacin. IMPORTANT: Taking doses of Niacin may cause your body to flush a bright red. This phenomenon, though startling, will subside shortly since all B-vitamins flush out with water.

LDL (bad) cholesterol level should be below 100 mg/dL. Doctors typically offer a patient whose levels are higher a Statin drug. These drugs have been known to produce strokes. Instead try some of the tips below for a month; take fish oil and lecithin daily. Ask to have a repeat test scheduled in a month; my spouse's results dropped below the appropriate level in that amount of time.

Tips to lower cholesterol: Take a fish oil capsule daily. Make sure the source is mercury-free; Take lecithin capsule(s) or granules; Eat whole eggs without fear (lecithin in the egg white counters any cholesterol in the yolk);

Limit your intake of commercially fried foods; Bake foods rather than fry. New air fryer appliances may allow you to eat your favorites without the grease; Limit sugary foods; the liver will convert excess sugar to cholesterol; Eliminate tropical oils from your diet; Drink green tea.

Liver Issues – Consult a doctor immediately. Pain in the middle of your body directly under the ribs could be related to liver issues. Here is a list of things, some minor and others major, that can cause liver discomfort:

Once the gallbladder is removed, a person's liver takes over some responsibilities and can store fat globules as the gallbladder once did. Always drink some fresh lemon juice after a greasy, fatty meal; lemon juice is the only natural substitute for bile. See Gall bladder information in Chapter 10.

Exercise that is strenuous and/or recent which your body is unused to can result in a change in your liver enzymes. This is usually temporary.

Detox tea or any other source of detoxing. Chemotherapy causes detoxification issues because of the many cancer cells that are killed off.

Alcohol in large quantities and drunk regularly, such as an alcoholic consumes.

IMPORTANT: Avoid Alcohol. Whenever your body is in detox mode—from exercise, food, drink or drugs—refrain from consumption of alcohol, even in small quantities. The liver purifies all blood that passes through the body to remove toxins. Alcohol makes its task more difficult.

Herbal Help for Liver. There is one herb that is known to maintain liver health: Milk Thistle. Shaklee offers a DTX product for liver health which includes Milk Thistle. I have taken that product for many years now. No discomfort since. IMPORTANT: Your life is dependent on a healthy liver.

Chronic Kidney Disease Diet. By age 72, the average person's kidneys operate at 25% of original capacity. A preventative diet should also include only foods recommended for your blood type. Read the Blood Type Diet section.

Maintenance Diet. Those with stage 3 or 4 renal disease must limit foods that contain the minerals potassium and phosphorus, found in whole grains, nuts, red meat and cheese. These minerals can undermine the kidneys' ability to keep you safe. Follow the dietary guidelines provided by a renal doctor or nutritionist.

Follow Others: Aging Wisdom from Beatitudes, Nature, Kinfolk

Kidneys cannot remove high phosphorus levels; extra phosphorus can pull calcium out of your bones.

If your potassium becomes too high, it can cause an irregular heart beat or worse. Most foods are high in potassium; even low potassium foods eaten in quantity can cause an issue.

Wheat is one of the biggest offenders, as are dairy and nuts.

Gluten Sensitivity Diet. This trendy dietary-related disease has stormed the American public. Celiac disease is the most sinister form of gluten sensitivity. The current crops of wheat, cultivated to produce many more and larger wheat kernels than in days gone by, are responsible for some of this problem. You may want to consider the purchase of products that use some of the ancient grains, such as Quinoa, Spelt, Barley and Kamut.

I attended a talk given by a local woman who was one of the first to package gluten-free mixes for baked goods. She admitted that her first trials didn't sell until she added sugar to them. This confirmed to me that sugar also contributes to Celiac disease.

Gluten Substitutes. You can now buy these prepared items in freezers and on grocery shelves in almost every store. Experiment until you find choices that taste good and/or cause fewer health issues than wheat-based products.

Bread—Millet bread; Rice flour; Spelt bread

Pasta—Corn; Rice; Lentil and other Veggies variations; spaghetti squash

Follow Others: Aging Wisdom from Beatitudes, Nature, Kinfolk

Cook with Healthy Grains. Packages of ground grains can be bought online or in almost every grocery store. If looking for something specific, check a health food store. Good cook books abound for baking with whole grains. Recipes tell how to bake everything from pastries to biscotti. Remember about the possible connection of sugar to Celiac disease.

Salt Sensitivity and Substitutes. If you are or become salt sensitive as you age, your blood pressure will rise and fall dependent on what you eat. I did not realize how much salt there is in tomato and its products. For an Italian, this came as quite a shock to me.

There are a few lower-salt soups and even tomato sauces. Regardless, you will have to make more of your own foods using these tips on non-salt substitutes. Mrs. Dash is a commercially prepared salt-free product. Or make your own substitute using recipes in the Quick Fix Healthy Mix cookbook by Casey Kellar and Nicole Keller-Munoz.

Spices can be used individually or select a combination suitable for the recipe type. Prepared substitutes are available at grocery stores. Sprinkle less aggressively than you would salt. Individual spice listing and recommended uses:

Turmeric—Chicken, Turkey and Lamb; rice

Paprika—Polish foods

Garlic powder—Italian foods

Onion powder—Hamburger

Celery seed—Veggie meals

Parsley flakes—Italian or Veggie

Poultry seasoning—Turkey and Chicken

Follow Others: Aging Wisdom from Beatitudes, Nature, Kinfolk

Mustard—Dry in meatloaf; use prepared mustard sparingly

Herbal Bouquet type—Meats

Pepper—Use ground black pepper sparingly; under the microscope it resembles shards of glass. Substitute Cayenne pepper in small amounts.

Water Drinkers. Water flushes toxins out of the body. Dehydration can cause you to feel lethargic with low energy. Here's a chart I found online of when it is important to drink water. Also drink water when feeling hungry between meals or resisting a virus.

Correct time to drink water per a Cardiac specialist:

2 glasses after wake up – helps activate internal organs

1 glass 30 minutes before meal – helps digestion

1 glass before a bath – helps lower blood pressure

1 glass before bedtime – avoids stroke or heart attack; prevents leg cramps

Water – Filtered and Bottled. There are several types of filters available to remove chemicals from tap water. Some attach to your faucet and others sit in your refrigerator. Or you can buy spring water; unfortunately for some they come in plastic bottles.

Kidney stones. Unfiltered water could result in kidney stones, if local water has a high ratio of calcium. Stick to bottled water if that is your local scenario. Passing a kidney stone is right up there in pain with childbirth. Dehydration is another cause of kidney stones as well as gout.

Follow Others: Aging Wisdom from Beatitudes, Nature, Kinfolk

Veggie/Fruit Flavored Water Substitutes. Can't tolerate the taste of plain water? Consider a pitcher with strainer insert. You can add tea bags, fruit, citrus or veggie ingredients to lightly flavor your water.

Sports Nutrition and Drinks—If you exercise regularly, you need to manage your protein, electrolytes and water levels. For information on Protein and Electrolyte drinks, read more below. Maximize recovery with a drink immediately after workout and again in two hours. Disclaimer: this information comes directly from the Shaklee website of which I am a distributor.

Protein Replacement Drinks. Types of protein drinks fall into several categories. All come with measurement scoops when adding to a liquid, such as milk, almond milk, water or juice. Choose the best one for you based on allergies, specific needs and sweeteners. Common sweeteners used are stevia (plant based), lacto-based (animal based). Flavors offered are typically Vanilla and Chocolate. Other flavors such as pumpkin, coffee and strawberry may be seasonal.

Whey Protein—Look for 100% grain-fed sources.

Soy Protein—Heart-healthy soy, with 9 essential amino acids. Soy lowers thyroid body temperature and may help with menopausal hot flashes. Those on beta blockers or blood thinners may want to avoid for that reason.

Vegetarian Protein—Vegan, gluten-free, kosher, keto-friendly

Follow Others: Aging Wisdom from Beatitudes, Nature, Kinfolk

Performance Drinks. To hydrate, mix in water or juice. For those exercising, place powder in empty water bottle, then add water and shake. To build lean muscles, mix in cold milk or water.

Ingredients may include: Green coffee – take before work outs or when a burst of energy is needed; Carbohydrates – take during exercise.

CAUTION: Caffeine energy drinks do not contain all the nutrients needed by the body for exercise. Always hydrate with water and or a prepared performance drink with many nutrients recommended for exercise.

End Point: "Well, you know I'm getting on." Getting on where? What do they mean, getting on? Do they want sympathy? We don't need to grow old and tired out, weary and discouraged. When you find God, you find life.

Prayer Point: Let the weak say, I am strong. Joel 3:10b

Follow Others: Aging Wisdom from Beatitudes, Nature, Kinfolk

Follow Others: Aging Wisdom from Beatitudes, Nature, Kinfolk

Beatitude: You are the light of the world. A city set on hill cannot be hid. Nor do men light a lamp and put it under a peck-measure [bushel] but on a lamp stand, and it gives light to all in the house. Let your light so shine before men that they may see your moral excellence and your praiseworthy, noble and good deeds and recognize and honor and praise and glorify your Father Who is in heaven. Matthew 5: 14-16 Amplified

Chapter 12—Motivation in Motion

Exercise in the pool is excellent for strengthening your CORE muscles. A simple exercise can be done while at home, even standing at a counter making supper or washing dishes. For this tummy tuck: suck in your stomach/abdomen and hold to the count of 30; then release. This can be done in tandem with Kegel exercises for bladder control. I just read an article that says wearing women's stretch pants weakens the CORE muscles. I'm guilty of that recently due to jeans bothering my hemorrhoids. Ouch, did I just admit that in public?!

Brain Health. Dr. Amen, a specialist on the brain, recommends exercise as one way to increase brain health. Consider these alternative ways to increase dopamine (mood altering):

Low value dopamine-producing activities or substances – caffeine, excessive screen/TV time, scary movies

High value activities that increase dopamine and strengthen the brain – exercise, massage, green tea, youth restorer supplements (see previous chapter).

Follow Others: Aging Wisdom from Beatitudes, Nature, Kinfolk

Exercise Untruths. Exercise is not what you do so you can eat whatever you want. While exercise provides a break from mental stress, only rest and massage removes the muscle knots created by stress. Exercise is not just an excuse to own and wear a fitbit-type tracker on your wrist.

Targeted Exercises. Chapters throughout this book mention exercises for specific areas of the body, such as the face, eyes, shoulders and hips. See the list below:

Chapter 6—Heart Health, walking, aerobic; Neck, tightening

Chapter 7—Eyes, series of eye motions; change focus; Jaw/TMJ, uniform facial stretches; Face/skin, massage

Chapters 7, 9—Incontinence, Kegel

Chapter 8—Shoulder/Bone Spurs, therapy; target exercise; Arthritis, moderate exercise; walking; Osteoporosis, load bearing; walking; Knees, therapy, stretches; Parkinson's Disease, water; Tai Chi

Chapters 8, 9—Hips, CD on hip exercises, posture

Chapter 9—Arms, tighten flabby arms

Chapter 12—Depression/Brain health, Exercise; massage

Gymnastic Adventures. For overall exercising suggestions, see Chapter 10.

Maximum Heart Rate. Related to age, this heart rate should not be exceeded during exercises. To calculate your max heart rate: Subtract your current age from 220, then multiple by 70 to 75%. For example, the max heart rate for those in their 70s is between 102 and 113. To test without a fitbit-type tracker or other monitoring device, place two fingers on your neck and count the number of beats in a minute.

Follow Others: Aging Wisdom from Beatitudes, Nature, Kinfolk

Cardiovascular/Heart Health. The heart is an organ about the size of your fist. Its pumping action is the work of four cavities and matched valves. The medical profession measures the blood pressures within the heart that pump blood through the cardiovascular system of veins and arteries.

Tips to improve heart health: Avoid stress; Reduce weight and cholesterol; Cut out salt (salt sensitivity) - lowers heart rate; Don't smoke– this will increase vitamin C availability; Reduce carbs – this lowers systolic number; Drink green tea; Beet powder or chews can raise blood pressure for some people

Blood Pressure – Consult a doctor immediately regarding high or very low. Doctors care most about the Systolic and Diastolic blood pressures. The ideal rate is 120/70. Acceptable numbers change as we age because blood vessels become less pliable.

The upper number (systolic) records the pressure when the heart is pumping. The lower number (diastolic) records the pressure while the heart rests between beats. The heart rate is a third number collected which provides information about how often the heart beats per minute. There are many factors that can affect these three rates.

Systolic Pressure Factors

Higher: Salt intake. Read labels; look for low-salt versions. Reduce tomato/products; White collar syndrome; Stress; Most cold remedies; Ibuprofen

Lower: Low potassium caused by low protein intake; Antihistamines; Olive Leaf Extract – reduced LDL and improved flow in blood vessels

Follow Others: Aging Wisdom from Beatitudes, Nature, Kinfolk

Diastolic Pressure Factors

Higher: High intake of carbs (pasta, bread, baked goods); Diabetes or pre-diabetes.

Lower: Beet powder – expands blood vessels to aid blood flow; Hawthorn Berry – anti-oxidant removes plaque that can build up and block vessels; Olive Leaf Extract – reduced LDL and improved flow in blood vessels.

Heart Rate Factors

Higher: Salt intake. Read labels and look for low-salt versions. Reduce tomato products; Hyperthyroidism with afib, palpitations; Having the flu or a broken bone can cause a high heart rate as the body tries to heal; sleep is the best remedy.

Lower: Hypothyroidism – increases with age; Atenolol, beta blocker.

Natural Tips for Heart Health:

Herbs: three herbs improve blood flow through blood vessels and decrease high blood pressures (see details in Blood Pressure section): Beet root; Hawthorn berry; Olive root extract.

Vitamins/Nutrients: CoQ10 increases youthful energy; see section earlier in the book; L-Carnitine increases oxygen supply to heart (see earlier Youth Restorer section); Magnesium needed with calcium for growth of bones.

Heart Related Diseases. The heart is an amazingly resilient organ, pumping 2000 gallons of blood every 24 hours. Factors that can affect heart health:

Follow Others: Aging Wisdom from Beatitudes, Nature, Kinfolk

Thyroid issues are an important and often overlooked factor.

Hardening of heart muscles due to prolonged high blood pressure

Aging blood vessels may restrict blood flow; herbs can improve blood flow through these vessels.

Other age-related factors that affect heart health are diabetes, obesity and cholesterol levels.

Low blood sugar, although not necessarily age related, can be triggered by Beta Blockers. Cut the tablet in half or take smaller amounts at both breakfast and night time. The blood sugar spikes and dips will be reduced in intensity.

Autoimmune diseases can affect heart muscle health, per Dr. Gundry author of the Longevity Paradox.

Stress can cause a skipped heart beat. This may be due to low vitamin D which regulates the heart's electrical system. More noticeable in winter when oily vitamins are sluggish.

Congestive Heart Failure – Consult a doctor immediately. This condition results from hardened heart muscles that make it difficult to pump fluids. The most notable symptom is holding fluid in the abdomen/lungs; this may require doctors to siphon off fluid and prescribe personal oxygen tubing. The end result of congestive heart failure is renal shut-down.

Oxygen Usage: Personal oxygen sources limit user travel. Ask your doctor for guidelines on oxygen usage.

Smoking- Related Diseases. Give up smoking tobacco to add years and improve quality of life in your senior years. I lost a dear friend who

Follow Others: Aging Wisdom from Beatitudes, Nature, Kinfolk

learned that lesson the hard way. Besides, quitting cigarettes can save money as well.

Carotid artery. Blockage of this artery in the neck region is typical of smokers. It is called COPD.

Emphysema. This disease of the lungs is typical of smokers. The lungs become so damaged that swallowing wrong could end in death.

Exercise by Body Type. Choose the type of exercise that helps nourish and support weaker glands as per recommended in Dr. Abravanel's body type diet book. Dependent on your strongest gland type, he recommends specific combinations of strength training, cardiovascular workouts, yoga stretches as indicated below. Our preferences for exercise tend to utilize only our strengths. See what not to do for each body type, and consider that those exercises might be perfect for you.

Adrenal type – need flexibility not strength; need cardiovascular like tennis, yoga, light weights; not heavy weight lifting which can damage hips

Gonad type – need strength, cardiovascular, yoga; NOT horseback riding, bicycling, skating

Thyroid type – need strength, cardiovascular, stretching, backpacking; NOT bicycle or tennis in short bursts

Pituitary type – need to integrate mind and body like aerobic dancing, strength, moderate cardiovascular, 5 minute yoga; NOT long distance running or rowing

Walking is excellent exercise for any body type. Refer to Dr. Abravanel's book for detailed exercise plans.

Follow Others: Aging Wisdom from Beatitudes, Nature, Kinfolk

Time of Day for Exercise. Unfortunately for many of us, the best time of day to exercise is mornings. What can you do if you are not a "morning" person?

Schedule a part of your exercise routine for early in the morning. I do my stretch exercises in the shower where the warmth loosens up tight muscles. I work on my shoulder therapy exercises then as well.

I try to use my elliptical trainer before the day begins, with some minor stretches before starting. Three hundred steps is my maximum. I ride my stationary bike in the late afternoon while watching TV reruns.

Walking can be done early, mid-day and evenings.

Training classes at a gym often run in the afternoon, and are good for those who exercise best in a group with music.

Perform exercises to strengthen Core muscles on the floor in front of the TV in the evening. Or put in a video on Tai Chi.

Gender Exercise Strengths. A trainer once told me that for men, their strength is in their arms; and for women, it is in their legs. The object of an exercise plan is not to overwork your strongest points at the expense of those weaker. We have seen women athletes who have marvelous musculature but little breast tissue left.

Find an exercise plan and time table that firms and tones you—body, soul and spirit. You will enjoy it the rest of your life.

Introvert/Extrovert. You may feel more comfortable exercising by yourself. Pool laps may be perfect for you. If you need companions, sign up for an aerobics class at a gym or town-operated facility. Or exercise listening to music.

Follow Others: Aging Wisdom from Beatitudes, Nature, Kinfolk

Low Impact Exercise. Because of repeated issues I've had with my shoulders, the average exercise classes can cause me to over-reach and irritate those joints. Here are some low impact exercises that may be available at your gym or pool.

Tai Chi. This low impact exercise helps seniors in many ways. These include better balance, sleep patterns, reduced stress and flexibility/coordination. Classes are good, or by DVDs may be the best way for seniors. If you are fortunate enough to have Tai Chi available in a pool, don't miss the chance to attend.

Swimming. Like walking, swimming is a universal low-impact, aerobic exercise. Repeat two or three times a week faithfully for improved health.

Ballroom Dancing. My sister and her husband in their fifties put in many hours on the dance floor. They attended and won competitions, dressed to the nines, with their dance instructors.

Silver Sneaker Program. If you can't afford to pay fees for gym access, find a Medicare Advantage plan that includes enrollment in the Silver Sneaker Program. At my gym, there is no charge if Silver Sneaker people wish to use the gym after 1 pm. If I want to exercise earlier in the day or use the pool, it costs me $10 a month. Very affordable, indeed.

House Work is Exercise. A friend's mother is 104 and she has always done all her own housework. I've been assured her house is immaculate. Aging people can and should count housework as exercise. A mileage tracker will let you know how many miles you walk daily. And just between you and me, I think I own the most heavy and

Follow Others: Aging Wisdom from Beatitudes, Nature, Kinfolk

difficult to use vacuum cleaner ever, though check out my muscles. Purchase of a lighter model might make house cleaning less of a chore.

CORE exercises. These exercises tighten the muscles of the abdomen. Firm core muscles stabilize the body and prevent the incidence of falls. These will help in rising and sitting down in a chair. See my CORE story at the beginning of this chapter.

Avoiding Falls. Suggestions to Stay Safe:

Never continue to exercise until you feel pain. Pain is not the goal of an exercise plan—not even for therapy sessions.

Research other options. Speak with a therapist or trainer at your local gym about activities that best suit your needs.

Don't stop exercising until your mind says to stop. Per fitness trainer and author, Marc T. Woodard.

Substitute Less Dangerous or Repetitive Exercise. Did you love ice skating, like a friend of mine who has had a stroke? Her doctor advises she not try ice skating again. Maybe cross country skiing or snow shoeing would provide the same winter weather adventure and exercise with less risk of falls.

I personally never took up jogging because of the likelihood of sports' injury, but I used to enjoy a quick sprint around my side yard followed by fast walking. I also like 3-minute sessions on the elliptical trainer set up in my laundry room.

Most important is to reduce the number of repetitions you were able to do while a youth. Also, reduce any weights used for lifting or while walking. This prevents injuries to joints caused by repetition.

Follow Others: Aging Wisdom from Beatitudes, Nature, Kinfolk

Equipment Needed. Prefer to exercise at home? Advantages are no driving and no monthly fees. Before buying equipment for home use, check into the Silver Sneakers Program mentioned above.

Weights—Care should be taken when weights are added to an exercise regime. Start with smallest weight and work up gradually. Recommended: 1 to 3 pound barbells

Ankle weights – smallest is best. I limped around after trying ankle weights without prior testing. Returned them to the store as soon as I could make it there.

Rubber Bands – These are the therapists favorite for shoulder issues. Color-coded for resistance provided. Start with yellow or green.

Mechanical Equipment – Watch Out. I own the first item listed below. Most items can be purchased from Target or other box stores; the elliptical trainer cost around $300.

Elliptical trainer – men may not appreciate the stride

Rower – may be too strenuous for certain body types (see above)

Stationary Bike – men who ride bicycles too often can experience prostate issues.

Treadmill – lets you run inside; however feet can get stuck in or slip off the moving track.

Braces – Once you reach Medicare age, you will start receiving phone calls about back and knee braces that can be supplied without charge to

Follow Others: Aging Wisdom from Beatitudes, Nature, Kinfolk

you. I haven't responded to one of those calls yet. But if you are on Medicare or Medicaid these benefits are probably available to you.

The goal of a brace is not to eliminate pain (read section on ointments for that), but to keep pain to a minimum so you can participate in activities and exercise with less difficulty.

NOTE: Do not act like a 20-year-old just because you are wearing a brace, unless you are a 20-year-old!

Healing Therapy and Therapists. Injured joints will not heal to full range of motion without therapeutic exercise. There are many types of therapies available. After surgery or major injury a doctor will recommend rehabilitation therapy such as described in the section on Shoulder and Knee Injuries.

Rehabilitation therapy. A portion of this therapy will be covered by Medicare or supplemental plans. Be sure to check what portion of this therapy is your responsibility to pay. In some states a doctor's script covers all charges; in other states the co-pay per visit is between $30-40. This adds up quickly if you need bi-weekly visits over a 13-week period.

Chiropractic/Acupuncture/Naturopath. Visits to a therapist who practices natural healing techniques can cost $50-80 a session. A company-paid insurance plan may cover the cost of limited visits. I have visited all three of these specialists, while trying to lower my blood pressure without medication. I might still visit an acupuncturist, as needed, for colds, TMJ and other tension-related issues. A single visit can produce health results that last for months.

Chiropractor. The chiropractor performs therapeutic manipulation of your spine and joints. This technique can be useful to relieve minor pain typical of the aging process and/or computer work. CAUTION:

Follow Others: Aging Wisdom from Beatitudes, Nature, Kinfolk

Avoid chiropractic manipulation if you have been diagnosed with osteoporosis or if you have a neck-related injury.

Acupuncture. The acupuncturist applies thin needles to meridian points on the body to help the body heal internal issues, cold and nasal issues and overall well being. This is most useful for widespread issues or those that are difficult to influence by manipulation. You may fall asleep the first session. Those who fear needles can rest assured that those used by the acupuncturist are extremely fine.

Naturopath. A naturopath uses homeopathic remedies to heal chronic and/or acute health issues. They may use other techniques, such as a colonic, to eliminate toxins from the body. The naturopath is an excellent source for homeopathic information. My doctor provided a class on how to use the remedies for acute and chronic situations.

Books on Homeopathy list symptoms/modalities for the most recommended remedies. Books are also available with specific information for infants/children; Homeopathic remedies are safe enough for children, too. My grandchildren and now great-grandchildren have all safely tried these remedies.

There is also a book for using homeopathy for muscular and skeletal healing. Recommended potencies are lower than 30c because of addressing deep body issues. See the Resources section for books recommended.

Massages that Heal. IMPORTANT: Use a gentle but firm touch when performing hand/feet reflexology.

Hand/Feet Therapeutic Massage. Reflexology therapy is based on mapping connections between the hands and feet with corresponding organs and glands of the body. Gentle massage of a foot or hand by

Follow Others: Aging Wisdom from Beatitudes, Nature, Kinfolk

someone trained in this therapy can help heal internal organs. For example, massaging areas down the side of the foot near the heel can help with issues in the colon. We had this massage done for my spouse while in the hospital with pancreatitis. Nowadays hospitals accept help from practitioners of natural health medicine.

Hand massage can target all of the endocrine glands to restore energy, or all sinus-related areas to release congestion. Specific internal organs can be stimulated. Reflexology graphics are available online. See the Resources section for books recommended.

Pain Erasure. Bonnie Prudden's Pain Erasure book demonstrates trigger point therapy is taken from. In general, Prudden's theory rests on the fact that when the body experiences injury in a specific area, such as legs, head/neck/back or torso, massaging a single trigger point closest to the injury can never relieve the pain. This is because of sympathetic responses from other trigger points in the area.

For example, if you bang your knee, trigger points in the calf, thigh and lower back will all be affected. Prudden's book shows all trigger points that need to be 'erased' and demonstrates how to do so. My chiropractic doctor and his family entertained the author in their home in Connecticut.

Cranial / Sacral Massage. My spouse suffered cranial injury in a crash initiated from behind by an 18-wheeler truck. He drove a Pontiac Fiero that was struck sideways and propelled into an adjacent lane. My spouse's head whiplashed and struck the speakers and support frame behind and on either side of his seat.

We pursued many therapists for relieve from the constant pain at the rear of his skull. To this day he cannot tolerate the pressure of a

Follow Others: Aging Wisdom from Beatitudes, Nature, Kinfolk

baseball cap or spring-loaded eye glass frames. At a local community college, we attended a training on Cranial/Sacral massage. The trick is to apply pressure to two opposing locations, but to only push in the direction that has less pain. From there we searched for a local a doctor practicing in the area. Since the skull has many interlinked bones, this condition took a while to stabilize. Some chiropractors attempted to use basic strategies, but there was little relief until several skilled practitioners used their skills. This must be done along with monitoring cranial pressure shifts. Consider this therapy for: Post-cranial trauma; Eye glass correction – (surprisingly pressure changes within the skull can be gauged to eliminate need for tri-focals)

Natural Ointments/Treatments. In general, infusions, tinctures, lotions are made by soaking healing herbs in warm water (infusion), in alcohol (tinctures) or in oil (lotions) for application to the skin.

Chinese Medicine. Practitioners may use an assortment of the following remedies:

Tiger Balm – external analgesic that uses menthol as active ingredient to reduce issue inflammation. This remedy also contains oil/herbal ingredients such as Peppermint, Cinnamon and Licorice

Stone therapy – use of heated stones to help the body heal

Cupping – alternative strategy using cups on the skin to create suction and promote healing, similar to deep tissue massage.

Homeopathy. Also see section on homeopathy basics later in this chapter.

Arnica Montana – muscle pain from injury; 30 c potency; Post surgery – order Arnica 200ck potency online; to help healing take a dose

Follow Others: Aging Wisdom from Beatitudes, Nature, Kinfolk

(several sublingual pills) whenever pain is noticed. This remedy is made from an herb is local in Montana; a co-worker from that state keeps a supply of the Arnica flowers for making her own infusions to soak an injury.

T-relief – injury to muscles and tendons. A combination of many homeopathic remedies, such as Arnica Montana, in low potencies to relieve pain. (dog tested)

Aromatherapy. I have little experience in this field due to being allergic to smells. However, I have successfully used the following essential oil combinations. If interested, research this methodology further online.

Muscle Ease by Nature's Truth- contains peppermint, rosemary, cinnamon leaf and Arnica (homeopathic).

Choose a product that is low in fragrance, for those with allergies. Use only a few drops of herbal oil in carrier oil.

Sports Medicine. Cold therapy pain relief sprays/creams – topical analgesic such as Biofreeze were standard for use on therapy patients; now advertised for sports-related pain.

Electrical muscle stimulation therapy – two electrodes applied to the body so current can flow between, used with cold compress to stimulate healing after therapy treatment. My personal favorite.

Menthol creams – Shaklee Footcream – analgesic creams applied to skin to reduce muscle/tendon pain

Heat vs. Cold Applications: Heat for middle back injuries/pain; Cold for extremities: shoulder/knee injury or recent surgery; Heat and then cold for recent injury and before therapy.

Follow Others: Aging Wisdom from Beatitudes, Nature, Kinfolk

My Kids, Food Hated and Still Remembered

As mentioned elsewhere in this book, I became interested in nutrition based on my own poor health. I now realize that this less related to hypochondria and more to my blood type A.

Since I was the cook, both at home and at my kid's school cafeteria, my four children served unwillingly as guinea pigs for my experiments with healthy food. I have to explain that in the 1970s there was very little information and/or recipes available about healthy eating. I knew a person whose kids had allergies and we passed a few recipes around. I started buying books that told me how to bake with natural ingredients after my third son called my birthday cake recipe "Concrete cake with Carob frosting." Worse yet, I didn't let my kids share in birthday fare other mothers brought to school. At that time we had no white sugar, period. Of course, their father ate what he liked when at work and it was probably full of sugar.

Another fiasco recipe, Tomato Aspic, is always mentioned at family gatherings when my early cooking is discussed. The aspic used unflavored gelatin, tomato juice and veggies. Our family rule was you had to eat one spoonful of anything. After my first bite, I decided not to eat any more. As the kids dutifully finished their plates, they noticed mine still had the dreaded aspic. I explained that I took my required one bite and could not gag the rest down. Astonished faces circled the table. Touché.

Thankfully, I gave up on concrete cakes and learned over the years how to make some quite palatable foods. Check out the recipes below

Follow Others: Aging Wisdom from Beatitudes, Nature, Kinfolk

Odd and Favorite Recipes

Peanut Butter Soup. Believe it or not, the entire middle school eaters gulped it down. Adding government issue Peanut Butter to a celery-based soup made a filling addition to lunch. Of course, at that time nut allergies were unknown.

Rye Pizza. Rye flour makes a hearty addition to wheat flour and rises equally well as standard pizza recipes. It was a repeated favorite at school; one boy actually asked me for the recipe (had to re-calculate for home usage). FYI, rye flour strengthens muscles; however, it is not gluten-free.

Flax Pita. This recipe is a more recent addition found in the Wheat Belly book. It make a fabulous sandwich wrapper out of flax seed, egg and spices, cooked in a microwave.

Quinoa for Breakfast. Two versions are equally yummy. One cooks quinoa, like oatmeal, and adds blueberries and almond milk. The other recipe uses cooked quinoa and nut butter to bake a hand-held soft treat. See recipes in The Daniel Plan book. Quinoa that is cooked in a pressure cooker is best for intestinal health.

Carob Cream Pie. I consider this recipe my first dessert triumph. The crust includes pecans and whole wheat pastry flour (or substitute other flours). The filling is pudding made from carob powder, coffee/substitute granules to taste like chocolate, thickening and your preferred type of milk. Whipped cream on top makes it special.

Kale Chips. Break kale leaves off hard stems into large bite-size pieces then sprinkle and toss with a bit of oil and spices such as salt/pepper, garlic powder and/or paprika. Bake on oiled sheet at 375 degrees until crispy. Toss once. Similar to recipe from Melissa d'Arabian of Food Network Channel.

Follow Others: Aging Wisdom from Beatitudes, Nature, Kinfolk

Eggplant Stew. Slice or cube veggies including onion, celery, carrots and eggplant. Add whole tomatoes, beef broth. Spice with honey, garlic, allspice, pepper. Simmer covered 30 minutes. Add macaroni and parsley. Top with grated cheese. This recipe came from my earliest research on healthy eating. Unfortunately, I've lost the book title and author's name.

Homeopathy Basics – the long and short version. I became interested in homeopathy about twenty-five years ago when my grandchildren were young. I learned about it for myself from a naturopathic doctor and then taught it to my family. I was familiar with herbs at that time but learned that homeopathy worked faster than herbs—twenty minutes as opposed to three days. With children that is especially important, as a child can quickly become ill. And they are less apt to be allergic than to herbs.

You can go online any time to find out all about homeopathy, but here is the condensed version of how it works.

NOTE: There is nothing mystical about homeopathy; it is simply a variation of taking herbs for healing which works much faster with your immune system.

Source of Remedy. In the UK, homeopathy remains more popular than western medicine; the British queen uses it all the time. And 19th century Americans, such as Ralph Waldo Emerson's wife, used it to treat simple health issues: their other option was doctors with leeches, vaccinations and surgery. So there is a long-time history of testing certain herbs and commonly-known substances to record the homeopathic reactions/results.

Books on homeopathy offer suggested remedies organized by the illness type and patient weaknesses. Remedies address health conditions that someone might want a doctor to treat, such as stomach ache, teething pains, cold with fever, sprained ankle. Thinking in

Follow Others: Aging Wisdom from Beatitudes, Nature, Kinfolk

reverse—if a noxious herb might cause vomiting, the homeopathic version of it would cause the same immune reaction. Noxious? No fear—you'll see in a minute!

How modern-day homeopathic remedies are created: by agitation of huge vats of pure water to which a small portion of a noxious substance is added. Extraction of samples and agitation in new vats of water occur repeatedly as many as 10 (10X), 300 (30C) or more (200C) times. Western medicine claims there can be nothing of the original substance left in the final vat. Apparently the water molecules recognize that the substance was present at some point. Workers prepare tiny bottles or tubes filled with sugar pills and add a few drops of liquid drawn from the final vat. The remedy is ready for distribution.

How to Administer. Homeopathic remedies work in much less time than herbs. Herbal preparations take days before the body musters an immune response. The correct potency of homeopathic remedy is placed under the tongue where the pill/tablet dissolves almost instantly (for infants and toddlers crush and add to water). The body's immune system responds within minutes, rather than days.

NOTE: Remedies are most effective if you haven't eaten or drank (even water) just before taking the remedy. Coffee and mint-flavor toothpaste can counteract the efficacy.

Which Potency to Take. The typical dosage is 2 or 3 pills of the best remedy placed under the tongue. If no relief is experienced in 20 minutes, try another dose of the same or a dose of the next best remedy. No fear of overdoses; these are tiny sugar pills.

6C or 12C—If the health issue is related to the muscular structure of the body, a low potency remedy (6C or 12C) may prove most effective.

Follow Others: Aging Wisdom from Beatitudes, Nature, Kinfolk

30C—If the issue experienced is related to something a general practitioner or internist might be consulted about (cold, skin rash, head ache), then 30c is the standard potency. This potency works both for new or seldom-experienced (acute) symptoms, as well as ongoing (chronic) or flare up (acute) symptoms.

1000C—Some symptoms require higher potencies and different instructions. For example: if someone highly allergic to poison ivy runs into the leaves, use a single dose of 1000C or higher.

200C—After surgery, a 200C potency of Arnica can relieve pain and promote healing. This potency can be repeated as needed for pain after trauma.

200C—If the person is not improved of an acute illness with a 30C potency of the best remedy, they can try a single dose of 200C.

For potencies 200C or higher, place 2 or 3 pills of the target remedy under tongue. Do not repeat or use a weaker potency for at least one week; this is due to best absorption, not because of a dangerous dosage. You can simultaneously use different 30C remedies to help sympathetic issues.

Which Remedy to Use. Even if you have a photographic memory, you need to own a book on remedies. All such books have indexes to search by name of remedy or condition and give appropriate dosage instructions. For example, a modality suggests which remedy to use if the patient has cough with or without a fever, or pain on the left side versus right side.

IMPORTANT: The modalities are most important to quickly find the right remedy. There are seldom any ill effects no matter which remedy is used. These are basically sugar pills.

Follow Others: Aging Wisdom from Beatitudes, Nature, Kinfolk

For Pets. Search online for homeopathic remedies safe for use on pets. Research and consider these and other products that are safe for pets and people.

Rescue Remedy (drops) for cats stressed by moves or lost feline friend.

T-relief for dogs of certain breeds that suffer issues with their hips; also good for aging animals. We know a friend who found amazing results for her two older dogs who had trouble jumping up to her bed. Many testimonials by dog owners can be found online.

Safety Disclaimer: the above explanations should not be taken as medical advice. Refer to the book you purchased, instructions on the remedy bottle, or advice from a homeopathic practitioner. Because homeopathic remedies are distributed via sugar pills or milk-lactate tablets, the Biggest Safety considerations are:

For children: a sugar rush from overdosing, even if the entire vial of pills is mistakenly consumed. My grandson called it the candy medicine.

For adults and children: failure to consult a doctor should the issue not clear up within a day or two.

CAUTION: Consult an emergency technician or hospital for life threatening issues. Homeopathic remedies can be used safely until the person can receive professional care.

IMPORTANT: Do not use a remedy if you have a known allergic reaction to the source herb/substance.

Recommended Homeopathic Kits. Kits contain an assortment of typically used remedies in 30C potency and can be purchased online.

Follow Others: Aging Wisdom from Beatitudes, Nature, Kinfolk

Or go to a health food store and purchase remedies similar to those listed below, then place in a travel-style zippered, clear plastic pouch. Carry a few remedies in a lunch box or purse while at work or shopping.

Arnica Montana—Muscle sprains

Belladonna—Fever with red cheeks; allergy/Rhinitis

Chamomile—Ear ache; tooth ache

Cantharis—Bladder/UTI

Euphrasia Officinalis—Eye irritation

Hepar Sulphuris Calcareum—Strep throat

Kali Bichromium—Sinus/Laryngitis/Bronchitis

Nux Vomica—Nausea

Phosphorus—Dizziness, headaches

Pulsatilla—Thick mucus from cold

Rhus Toxichodendron—Joint pain; Poison Ivy

*There are other remedies you may want to consider. Refer to a book or ask a knowledgeable sales person at health food store.

Best-known Remedies. Most homeopathic remedies can be purchased from a health food store or online. Boiron is a major distributor of the remedies. Two popular remedies can be purchased in drug stores and grocery stores as well. These are:

Oscillococcinum is a flu remedy sold in the OTC cold sections of drug stores and grocery stores. The dosage is to take the entire contents of

Follow Others: Aging Wisdom from Beatitudes, Nature, Kinfolk

one tube immediately on first flu symptoms. Lie down or rest for a while, too.

T-Relief is a group of products whose major homeopathic ingredient is Arnica Montana. This remedy is made from a mountain daisy that grows in Montana and is known for its healing properties. I met someone from Montana who makes her own infusions from herb she has transported East to where she works.

IMPORTANT: Do not take if you are allergic to the herb, Arnica Montana.

As opposed to pain medicines, Arnica helps heal injured areas, and thus relieves the pain from healing. Arnicare products are distributed in gel or cream forms for surface application to injured muscles.

T-relief is a combination of remedies that can be taken orally whenever a topical application would not suit the injury.

Follow Others: Aging Wisdom from Beatitudes, Nature, Kinfolk

Specific Remedies

Rhus toxicodendron – anti-poison ivy; use the highest potency available as a prevention or cure.

Chamollia – Teething, Colic This information is great for grandmothers who are babysitting their children's children. To administer: Crush two 6c or 30c sugar pills and add to liquid, yogurt or applesauce. The lower potency (6c) has greater affinity to structural issues such as teeth and bones.

Babies' teething issues are often exacerbated by calcium deficiency. Sucking hurts gums so they can't get the liquid nourishment they thrive on. Ways to supplement calcium:

Spoon some yogurt fresh from the refrigerator into their mouths. Let them bite the spoon, the yogurt will still get into their mouths.

Give them a crushed chewable calcium-magnesium tablet such as from Shaklee.

End Point: In Appendix A, read my personal list of homeopathic and herbal remedies used to ward off winter-time illness, including colds and flu.

Prayer Point: Beatitude according to Luke—Woe unto you that laugh now! for ye shall mourn and weep. Luke 6:25b

Follow Others: Aging Wisdom from Beatitudes, Nature, Kinfolk

Follow Others: Aging Wisdom from Beatitudes, Nature, Kinfolk
Part 4: Life Changes

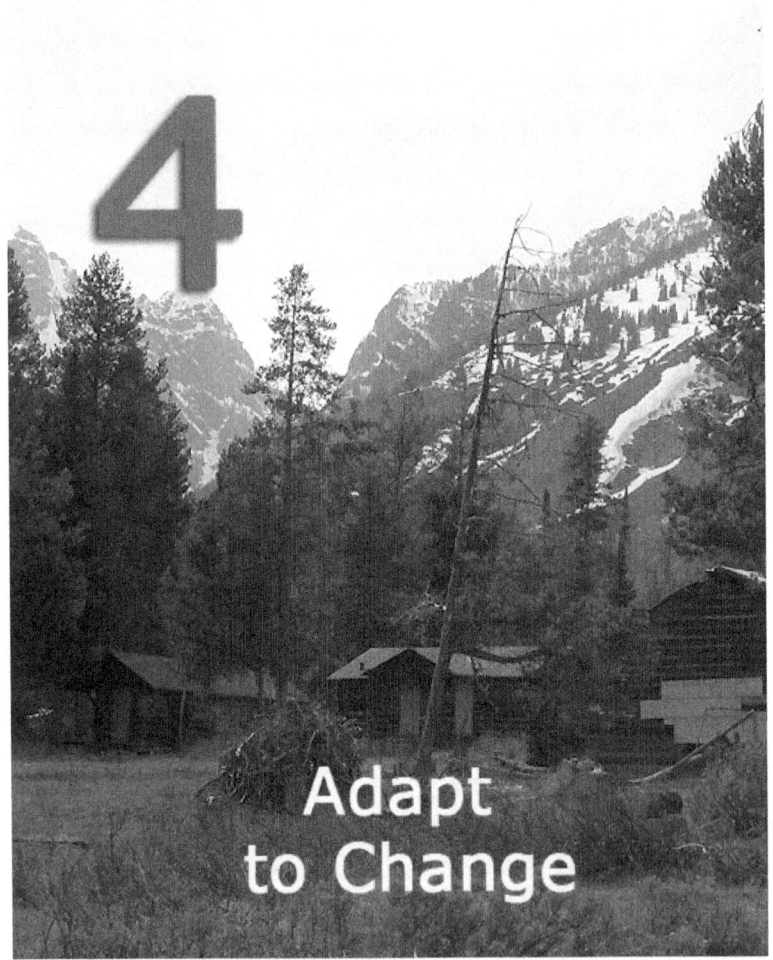

In This Part...

Chap13: Map Out Financial Plan

Chap14: Tough Choices – Push to Top

Chap15: Afterword

Follow Others: Aging Wisdom from Beatitudes, Nature, Kinfolk

Beatitude: ...being mindful of the words of the Lord Jesus, how He Himself said— It is more blessed—makes one happier and more to be envied— to give than to receive. Acts 20:35 Amplified

Chapter 13—Map Out Financial Plan

Many years ago I read about the life of Amy Carmichael, missionary to India. She helped rescue woman and girls threatened by society in both Britain and India. The story goes that her mother was worried about Amy being in the unseemly parts of town trying to raise money for a building where she could preach to the street "girlies." A friend of her mother advised: "God takes care of that kind of girl." I too have felt His Benevolent hand in providing for me despite my financial weaknesses.

Let's have a quick recap of the beatitudes as covered in the early chapters of this book. Remember that these were given as rules for the kingdom Jesus was about to set up. When we link with a king, won't we share in financial blessings as well?

Only you can decide how to spend or save your money. My suggestions are not the typical financial strategies given by a financial advisor. These are meant to expand upon methods that have already worked for you, with spiritual principles and senior discounts you may not have considered.

You'll be surprised to know that well-known financial gurus typically end their books with a chapter on Giving!

Beatitudes – Financial Rewards. Earlier we divided the beatitudes into two areas. Now, consider how the traits produced by living the beatitudes can bring financial rewards in each area.

Follow Others: Aging Wisdom from Beatitudes, Nature, Kinfolk

Inspiration for Life:

Grit – determination to achieve

Courage – fears/roadblocks removed

Enthusiasm – God breathed help

Confidence – able to carry on, to expect good things

Hope – not ashamed

Traits Worthy to Pass On:

Content – grateful

Compassionate – generous

Cooperative – work with others to succeed

Companion of Faithful Witnesses – serve others to gain blessings

Give Cheerfully. Have we found another of Jesus' beatitudes tucked away in the book of the Acts? When the Apostle Paul bid a final goodbye to the elders of Ephesus, he attributed this verse to Jesus. One may wonder why it is not mentioned in the book of Matthew with the other kingdom rules. Perhaps this one beatitude would have been unnecessary in the kingdom that Jesus first promised. If his hearers had kept the kingdom rules then, wouldn't everyone already have their needs met? Rejection on the cross, meant that Jesus' kingdom would have to wait. Instead, giving became the chief rule of blessing for this era—both Jew and Gentile.

Follow Others: Aging Wisdom from Beatitudes, Nature, Kinfolk

The Tithe. Left over from the Jewish nation who were required to give 10% to their religious leaders for temple maintenance. Does this mean that the tithe is no longer applicable? And didn't Jesus promise his followers blessings rather than request financial contributions? TV evangelists are criticized for their requests.

The tithe is less about who gets the money and more about who gets the greater blessing. In Malachi, the Lord promised that those who bring tithes into the storehouse will have a window opened in their lives, with blessing poured out, too much to store. This last phrase shows that the blessings received are to share with others.

Financial Advisors' Secret. Two books that I read on financial prosperity revealed a secret to financial success. Each author hid this gem away in their final chapter: give a tithe if you want to prosper. They did and became famous. Read the books by Suzie Orman and Richard Kowaski, Rich Dad, Poor Dad.

Charitable Gift Annuity. Charitable organizations, like those you may currently donate part of your tithe to, can provide advice on how you might set up an annuity. Read the Charitable Gift Giving sectionat the end of this chapter.

Other Half of Cheerful Gifts. A cheerful giver always sees oneself with enough, and a spare. It is the wonder of a full cup and what can be done with the portion not needed. I have been a cheerful giver most of my life. Whether this is a spiritual gift, a natural talent or both I cannot say. I do know, that some of my favorite memories are of times I gifted another person.

Gifts made by others also impress me. Do you remember the year that actor Bill Cosby and his wife, Camille, donated $20 million dollars to Spelman College in Atlanta? I do. It was 1988, near Christmas time. After unemployment and low paying jobs, our family of six did not

Follow Others: Aging Wisdom from Beatitudes, Nature, Kinfolk

have much money for celebration. Just as Nehemiah's sadness about the condition of Jews at Jerusalem was noticed by king Artaxerxes, my feelings must have shown on my face. My spouse questioned me, "Are you jealous of the sapphire pendant your sister received?" Totally surprised, I could only blurt out, "No. I'm jealous about not having a million dollars to give away."

For a person who enjoys giving, you might expect that Christmas is my favorite time of year. Actually, negative childhood events associated with the holiday left me rather bahumbug…until a magazine article caught my attention. The author suggested that holiday joy would come from a special gift to oneself—a present at Christmas time. This novel idea captivated me! And what gift would I enjoy most? Giving, of course, which for more than twenty years has become my annual present to myself. What a pleasure it is to decide on a mildly-extravagant dollar amount and then surprise an unsuspecting co-worker or acquaintance. It could be with a new coat that she would never buy herself, or a new bicycle just right for his daughter turning eight. The joy and wonder in their eyes shines brighter than any wrapped package under the tree.

Tithe Made Easy. As a cheerful giver, even tithing has come easy for me. With God, I cannot lose. He promises in the book of Malachi that He will open up the windows of heaven and pour us out a blessing. Why should I not believe that? Just so, , my family has experienced His provision in several seasons of unemployment. Rather than unemployment being a deterrent to giving, it simply reveals more gifting opportunities for the next time of employment…which, by the way, has always come. Until you personally have been there, you can never appreciate two bags of groceries left anonymously on your back porch or a $250 check placed in your hand to keep your child in day care.

Follow Others: Aging Wisdom from Beatitudes, Nature, Kinfolk

Receive Graciously. I was not aware that one could miss out on any part of giving until one summer in the late 1970s. My former Sunday School teacher and his family came to our church for a visit. He and his wife were on missionary furlough from Hawaii and stayed at our Vermont home for several days. They had adopted a bright Japanese boy from the islands who travelled with them. My teacher and his wife regaled us with tales of island life…where tropical showers are a part of each day and where their blond, blue-eyed daughters had been the racial minority in Hawaiian schools.

One morning I offered to show my teacher and his family the way to my Great-Uncle's home. Uncle Val and Aunt Letha (you met them earlier) lived at the top of one of the winding gravel roads that are the scrawled signature of rural Vermont. While in route, my Sunday school teacher reached out his hand. There was a $20 bill in it and he indicated this was for my kindness to his family. I was too surprised to even choke out the intended refusal. "It is my duty to provide for him, a missionary, and not vice versa," I stubbornly reasoned. Once more, my body language said what I could not.

The authoritative teacher's voice had not changed much since I was a skinny preteen. He countered my reluctance with these simple words. "Donna," he spoke patiently, "you have to learn to be a gracious receiver." I took the folded bill and mumbled a quick thanks.

In the years since that summer morning, his few words have echoed throughout my life. That short sentence was one he clearly learned at personal cost. What must it be like to always be at the receiving end, as missionaries and their families are? How must it feel to always depend on others' generosity, or lack thereof, to meet one's needs? This servant, who did the Lord's work in the Lord's way, deserved more respect than I had understood.

Follow Others: Aging Wisdom from Beatitudes, Nature, Kinfolk

My soul searches continued. Since the Bible states that it is more blessed to give than to receive, I wondered how many times this cheerful giver selfishly grabbed the greater blessing and embarrassed the recipient? And was there a time I gave publicly in order to receive recognition when an anonymous gift would have pleased the Lord more?

In a God-inspired turn of events that summer day in Vermont, the gifts (plural) given and received were multiplied by the greatest Giver of all. My teacher was blessed for his gift of $20 dollars. As the receiver, I was doubly-blessed with money—and with wisdom about gracious receiving.

Pass It Along. A few years later I had the first opportunity to pass my lesson learned on to another giver. This came as the result of a $54 gift to a Christian acquaintance whose husband had been diagnosed with cancer of the spleen. She was just as taken aback by my gift as I had been that morning in the missionaries' car. Her reason for surprise even surprised me. I had not known that she was the daughter of a millionaire. And her husband owned a lucrative business, which just happened to be a junkyard. My gift may indeed have been this rich person's first opportunity to receive graciously. Not to be outdone, she presented me with a hand-pieced quilt. The bonneted-ladies quilt graced my daughter's twin bed for years.

Now whenever I give to an individual, my teacher's words are always included as part of the gift. Also included is the suggestion that they should pass the money on when an opportunity presents itself. I hope, in this manner, to ease any embarrassment and to plant a crop of future givers.

Then I watch to see what blessings He, who was the first to give, pours out—until the cups of both the cheerful giver and the gracious receiver are filled and overflow.

Follow Others: Aging Wisdom from Beatitudes, Nature, Kinfolk

But my God shall supply all your need according to his riches in glory by Christ Jesus. Phil 4:19

Always Enough to Meet Needs. Whenever I feel pressure as a freelancer or contractor when my temporary income evaporates, this is what I say out loud to myself. Whenever I talk with someone who struggles financially, I quote this paraphrase to encourage them to believe the impossible, also. This favorite verse was written by the Apostle Paul to the Philippians:

I especially favor a paraphrase I picked up somewhere along the way. It goes like this: I always have enough to meet my needs and to give to others. Some people object to saying things that are not currently true. How can I say I have enough when I really don't? In a recent Joyce Meyer magazine, one article said it is like Jesus showing up at Lazarus' grave. The facts were that Lazarus was dead and buried. The Truth stood outside the door and he spoke: "Lazarus come forth." That specific dead man came back to life.

Financial Plateau. I learned of a financial concept while listening to a taped motivational talk given to me by a Shaklee sales supervisor. The speaker equated our current financial earnings to a plateau. He challenged that we reach a level of income and stay there until we make a commitment to progress higher. To prove this he asked his audience to compare tax returns for several years and see whether their earnings had reached a plateau. My husband had lost his fulltime job and we both were forced to work part-time jobs to supply our family of six. We lost our home to the bank, moved to a new state staying with relatives until we found more dependable work. This would be the perfect test of the plateau theory.

Here are the results as I remember them:

Follow Others: Aging Wisdom from Beatitudes, Nature, Kinfolk

Year my husband worked full-time at bank; me part time school cook = $22,000

Year my husband and I worked 3rd shift at temporary jobs = $22,000

Year my husband collected unemployment and I worked part time job in new state = $22,000

Needless to say I was amazed. And as soon as I realized the theory was true, I began to expect our income level to rise rapidly. I didn't document the next years but even in 1984, $22,000 was ridiculously low to support a family of six.

That third year, I remember someone asking me what my earnings were and I replied $12,500. When told that was way too little, I made a commitment with myself to prove their judgment of my potential earnings wrong. With a job change, within a few years I managed to quadruple my salary to $50,000.

Invest in Youth. Seniors have a great opportunity to invest in our young people. In the 1950s my father had to borrow from his brother the down payment for his first house. The amount was only $900 but it stood between my father and his lifetime personal goal. Interestingly, with the purchase of this home, my father who struggled with alcohol addiction never touched another drop. He had something of value to lose.

Now it is our generations turn to make the first-time home purchase a possibility for our grandkids. Some ways to assist financially:

Rent out space in your home without charge; better yet collect a small rent and deposit it in a savings account for when they are ready to buy. Make it legal with a contract.

Follow Others: Aging Wisdom from Beatitudes, Nature, Kinfolk

Advise them to get a second job, and perhaps speak a good word for them with an employer, church member or neighbor you know.

Offer each grandchild a sum of money when they make their first house purchase. We should all be able to give them $500, at least. My in-laws gave us $5000.

Buying that Last Car. Please don't ever say that this will be your last car. You might live another twenty-five years and have to purchase at least one more. To make a wise choice:

Compare prices online vs. a local dealership.

Buy last year's model in the fall.

Buy a car that gets low mileage and is large enough to provide access suitable for those with a cane.

Buy a second hand car if you or a relative are handy with maintenance.

Look into discounts available for car insurance from Fifty+ associations in next section.

Follow the guidelines for buying a car that is orthopedically appropriate for your body frame.

What NOT to do:

Don't forget to ask a mechanical friend to come with you.

Don't buy based solely on the color of the car.

Don't forget to pray before buying a car; only God can recognize a lemon.

Follow Others: Aging Wisdom from Beatitudes, Nature, Kinfolk

Senior Discounts – More Advantages and Some Adventure. Years ago the only way you could identify senior discounts was by buying a book as per advertised in some mailing. Nowadays, online searching makes it faster, and hopefully cheaper, to buy everything from a sandwich to life insurance.

The best senior discounts are ones that you use regularly or those that save money on expensive purchases like cars, insurance plans, eye glasses/lens and, of course, travel cruises.

National Associations. Fifty+ associations offer a multitude of discounts. For many years there was only one choice. We have to give AARP credit for not letting the grass grow under their feet, even without a rival. The moment someone hits that 50th birthday the AARP magazine arrives in your mailbox.

AARP is only one Option. Go online to their website to view member benefits by category. Or download the PDF list of membership benefits which makes it easier to compare between the new conservative fifty+ association. https://www.aarp.org/

AMAC option for conservatives. This organization, Association of Mature American Citizens, was created in 2007 to provide an alternative to AARP who supports less conservative values. The list of benefits was impressive as newcomers to the game. Since only discounts used are of any real benefit, you may want to do an online comparison before deciding which association to join based on benefits. I just printed a coupon for Friendly's that gives a free entrée with one purchased entrée. Here in New England Friendly's are neighbors; I visited the original in Wilbraham, MA as a teen. https://amac.us/

Follow Others: Aging Wisdom from Beatitudes, Nature, Kinfolk

Another list of senior discounts is available free from The Senior List. Check for your favorite restaurants and retail stores; many seem to be located in the southern states. Percentage discount, age requirements, and dates available make this list a useful tool. https://www.theseniorlist.com/biggest-list-of-senior-discounts/

Social Security, Medicare. Next year will you turn 62? If you have decided to retire early or just want to sign up for Medicare, make your appointment at a local Social Security office up to three months early.

Of course, you may try to enroll online—unless like my spouse you discover that someone else already tried to claim your SS card. That means he must contact in person to make changes to his status, hence the need for making an appointment three months ahead.

If you will turn 67, you can decide whether or not to claim your Social Security benefit. The SS recommends anyone still employed to wait until they turn 70. The fact is that the sooner you sign up, the more money you will eventually draw out of the system you've paid into for years.

Facts about SS:

If you collect Social Security (SS) at 62—you are limited to how much additional income you can earn without paying a penalty above a certain amount ($16,000). And of course, you may have to pay taxes on SS income dependent on your other income.

If you collect SS at 66 (or full retirement age)—you may continue working with no penalty for extra income. You may have to pay taxes on that amount depending on your other income.

If you start SS at 66—you could see your monthly amount increase if still working and earning at a higher salary than in the past.

Follow Others: Aging Wisdom from Beatitudes, Nature, Kinfolk

When you turn 70—the monthly amount becomes static, except for rate increases SS pays across the board to all recipients.

The cost of Medicare part B is withdrawn monthly from your check. This cost can increase depending on Medicare decisions. Medicare does not automatically cover part D for prescriptions. You must pay for it or join a Medicare-related plan that offers that coverage. See the next section.

Medicare Deadlines. CAUTION: Make appointments to sign up for Medicare three months before you turn 65. Otherwise, you may be charged a monthly late enrollment penalty for Medicare Advantage plans.

Health, Dental and Vision Insurance. Each fall companies that offer Medicare related insurance have open enrollment. Of course, if you qualify mid-year, you are allowed to enroll in a program without waiting. You can save very large amounts on premiums, deductibles and co-pays by shopping around. And good news, you don't have to do all of the research yourself.

Every state has a local association that will advise you of the best options based on your needs/circumstances. You may get a call from that association; if not, online research will help find their contact information. Also, large corporations such as Hewlett Packard provide this free advice service for retirees who qualify for Medicare.

These agents draw a commission based on how many of their referrals sign up for a given plan. The commission is not paid by you. So take advantage of this service, if you are unsure of your best options. They could help save you thousands of dollars over the yearly period. If not satisfied, you can switch insurance plans when the next renewal period rolls around.

Follow Others: Aging Wisdom from Beatitudes, Nature, Kinfolk

Types of Medicare insurance plans:

Medicare Advantage—This plan becomes the primary payer of your claims, even though you have Medicare. Some plans have Zero monthly payments. Some of these plans offer vision and dental benefits.

Gap programs—This type of Medicare-related plan begins to pay at the point you have met your deductible. It will pick up the remainder of charges for the current year.

Supplemental Insurance—This type of plan is often available while you are still employed and do not qualify for Medicare. It covers expenses incurred once you have met your employer-provided insurance deductible. The charge is minimal and billed to you directly. Claims must be submitted directly by you along with paid receipts.

Vision Benefits. If you don't have an insurance plan that covers vision, the optometrist and lens store can deduct a discount based on a membership, such as AAA. Check the discounts offered by a Fifty+ association as well.

Military Associated Benefits. Did you serve in the military? If so, there are special assistance and benefit programs that you may qualify for when your health begins to fail.

VA Benefits. Ex-military members who retired with honorable discharge are eligible to receive services at a Veteran's Administration hospital. If your case requires expertise, such as orthopedic doctor for hip replacement operation, VA can refer you to an outside doctor. Be prepared that times to make appointments may take longer than for a non-VA authorized doctor. https://explore.va.gov/health-care

Follow Others: Aging Wisdom from Beatitudes, Nature, Kinfolk

Aid and Attendance. For War era Vets 65 plus and their spouse, look into the benefits available to provide home or nursing home assistance. There is no savings monetary limit and you can own a home. However, the person must not be able to drive. Check this link: http://americanveteransaid.com/aid-attendance-benefit/

Leave Things Behind. It takes humility to leave any of the important things behind. What if you are not a humble person, you just can't afford to retire or you must have your independence in order to get to weekly bowling competition? And such changes are seldom voluntary.

"Forgetting those things which are behind..I press toward the mark for the prize of the high calling of God in Christ Jesus." Apostle Paul to the church at Philippi. Phil 3:13-14.

The Apostle Paul experienced the same things you and I must face or already have. Paul was aging with eye issues and travelled frequently, on foot, between churches he planted in Greece and in Asia Minor. He was stoned and nearly died several times for preaching the Gospel wherever he went. Soon he would be placed under house arrest for years in both Jerusalem and Rome. And a martyr's death awaited him. Now, that's involuntary changes!

Retirement. The ideal scenario is that you and your spouse both decide to retire at the same time so you can travel around the world in a newly-purchased RV home. You both participated in fantastic 401K programs and can manage well with a yearly income of $120,000. If lucky, your former employer offered insurance coverage for life.

My retirement was not like that; probably neither was yours. Yet I consider what actually happened to me is nearly as miraculous. I was early-retired in 2012. Here's how it happened. On the last Friday in

Follow Others: Aging Wisdom from Beatitudes, Nature, Kinfolk

May I was told about forced retirement coming; for good or bad measure, I was laid off the next Monday. Double-whammy. I was so annoyed that I threw my resume up online that day. Funny thing—the Lord had a job for me by the end of the week. Yes, it was contract, not full-time employment. With my two severance packages, from lay off and two months later early retirement, I netted the equivalent of an entire year's salary. Adding this income to the 5-month contract pay, my earnings doubled for the year of 2012, and nearly threw me into a higher tax bracket.

Lost company insurance forced me to apply for Medicare. I was already collecting Social Security. With two-years paid insurance and enough in savings, I could start a coveted second career as an author.

Forced Retirement. Read the issues and pluses of retirement based on temperaments at the end of this chapter. Forced retirement also teaches us the following values:

Being content where God has placed us at any given moment.

Submitting oneself to being second in command; consider the Apostle Peter who had to go where others took him when he was old.

Accepting work limitations that may result from surgery or falls.

Lost Job Means More Options. Don't take aging personally. Everyone will age, even that young upstart/college graduate who got your job. Now is the time for adventure, to give ourselves wholly to the hobbies and dreams we once held dear. Reread chapter 10 and find a thrilling new future for your final days.

Follow Others: Aging Wisdom from Beatitudes, Nature, Kinfolk

Move Away. "..the pursuit of home has become the pursuit of God—because I need to know that peace and rest can be found in every place I am, that there is reason and rightness beneath the chaos of my days." From author of Almost There.

You may be attached to the abode you and family have called home for ten, twenty or more years. You will miss the associations and affiliations shared over years. Bekah DiFelice moved repeatedly with her husband over his nine years in the Marines. In her book Almost There, she suggests that home doesn't begin or end with the mailing address or change in surname. The good news is that we never arrive to empty rooms empty handed. Amen.

With thirty-eight moves in my own life, I can vouch for the fact that we remake our own homes with the presence of those we love and the help of our loving God. New neighbors and opportunities add the sparkle we expected might be lost.

Down-size. Do you love to watch the Tiny House TV programs? I do and here is the reason why. I have moved many times in my life. I know how to down-size and pack better than any TV show host. First thing you do is plan a Tag or Yard Sale. An Estate Sale is appropriate if you are liquidating a parents' home and not your own.

Planning for the sale must include sorting current household and garage possessions into four 'piles' of items; those to: Keep to move or store; Sell; Give away; Trash.

Be aggressive, as once the sale starts it is often too late to include items you should have added earlier. My father-in-law found that out when I ran his first tag sale. They later had to donate a lot of things that would have sold well at the time.

Follow Others: Aging Wisdom from Beatitudes, Nature, Kinfolk

My Moving Story - New State with Newborn. My husband was laid off from his bank job only days before our third son was born. We had promised my aging VT family members (you met them earlier) that we would move up to help with the small church. Now, those promises were called in. We had to vacate the apartment we rented before Charlie could look for work. So we moved all our possessions into my Great Aunt and Uncle's apartment above the church— along with my sister's family; her husband had injured his arm and moved north before us.

I set up my first tag sale in the small back yard of our two-family apartment building. I'm sure I posted signs, but we were situated behind a local market, near Dunkin Donuts, and just off Center street at a main intersection. Location, Location, Location.

One of my mother's younger brothers came along to see what a Tag sale was like. Mine was the first this Uncle ever visited. He was amazed that I was selling so many nice things for such low prices. That's the name of the Tag Sale game.

Regrets, oh yeah! I wish I had kept the 8-place setting Noritake dinner set my husband brought back after stationed in Korea. And likewise the pearl ring he had purchased, which would have perfectly suited our daughter (not born at the time).

But we did sell enough to cover the expense of a moving truck with enough money left over to pay rent on our first residence in Vermont. And yes, my husband was hired by another bank—mainly because I was a native Vermonter and they only hired 'local boys.'

Plans for Financial Future. Many of us dread this financial task more than any required through youth and middle age. This is probably due to the universal dislike of considering our own mortality. As illustrated

Follow Others: Aging Wisdom from Beatitudes, Nature, Kinfolk

below what most of us dread can easily be checked off this particular to-do list.

Wills / Estate Plan. With the unexpected diagnosis of diabetes and Prostate cancer*, my former husband decided it was time to meet with a lawyer. Our eldest son accompanied him on several visits. Then they scheduled a meeting to sign the papers at the family house with all four siblings attending.

*Fortunately, test results show that the cancer is of treatable size and contained. Phew!

A complete package purchased from a lawyer can cost less than $500. This is what can be purchased for that price:

Quick claim deed – makes his children owners of the home, with agreement that their father can continue to live in the house.

Medical living will – designates which child/children are to make final hospital decisions. Any family doctor will be glad to provide you with a form to complete, as well.

Power of attorney – for paperwork signatures related to probate.

Executor of the estate – for probate issues, they decided to share responsibility between oldest son and only daughter.

Yes, much of the needed paperwork is available online. However, a lawyer can make paperwork for any complicated issue, like divorce, much simpler. And that fee includes work of a notary.

Church Gifts. A charitable gift annuity provides two benefits: ongoing income from your retirement funds and ability to name an organization as the beneficiary. This is an excellent idea for individuals/couples without children.

Follow Others: Aging Wisdom from Beatitudes, Nature, Kinfolk

Contact your favorite charitable organization about how to set up an annuity with their Financial Planning department.

Flora G, Mother of Faith

How many of us would willingly walk in the hard-working shoes of our relatives, especially the women? Flora Amelia was the middle child of her mother's second marriage. We met Achsa Amelia Corliss earlier. At sixteen my grandmother Flora met the love of her life, Bert G; they married that year. Bert was of Scottish descent with relatives on the Mayflower. He worked as a lumper in a granite shed in Barre, VT.

Mother of Ten. My grandparents had ten children. Flora bore three sons, then three daughters (my mother, Florence Amelia, was the middle daughter) and finally four sons only a few years apart. I was introduced to this family of ten children during World War II when my mother returned home to await my birth and my father's return from the war. You may have guessed my middle name is Amelia (likewise for my daughter and granddaughter whose story is told in Chapter 5); this tradition is strong in our family.

Everyone loved my grandfather (you'll meet him in the next chapter). Unfortunately Bert died early of hardening of the arteries. Flora was left with four young sons, the oldest, Jesse tall at 18 and three between 14 and 11 years old.

She was a praying woman who knew the Lord Jesus as her source, defender and strength. Once the boys got to the high school years, they joined the driving and drinking crowds in the evenings. They tell of going out to party and seeing her down on her knees in prayer. If you don't think that silent witness was of value, think again. Each of my uncles now has a relationship with their mother's Savior.

Follow Others: Aging Wisdom from Beatitudes, Nature, Kinfolk

Teacher of Girls. If you suppose Grandma Flora forgot how to train girls to become respectable young ladies after years of raising boys, you're mistaken. I apparently was the first granddaughter she got to practice on—a stubborn one in her eyes.

The first lesson she gave me was how to sew on a button. I was eight years old, but my mother was too busy to teach me, having children and dealing with our alcoholic father's issues. Always excited to learn, I sat near Grandma copying her motions. I may have noticed she was a bit prickly, having to travel to CT to watch me and my sister, but I was just proud of my new skills.

The second lesson she gave me was how to dress appropriately for the occasion. Out in the barn helping my uncle, I wore pants that nowadays we would call jeans. When asked if I wanted to drive into town, I climbed in the back seat without a moment's pause. The car followed the winding gravel road down to Montpelier —what I considered a small town (I lived in Hartford, CT and only vacationed in VT). I jumped out of the car happily, until Grandma spotted those dreaded barn pants. Boy, did I learn about the appropriate attire for certain occasions! It's a lesson I still remember, careful to check my appearance before any trip out of the house—even before using Zoom for online conferences.

Teacher of Words. When I learned to write poetry in school, I was told that Grandma too had written poems, a talent shared by many of her lineage. Recently on Facebook some of my cousins and siblings discussed colloquial phrases we picked up from Grandma. Funny how we each remember variations that pinned together make a colorful, colloquial whole. My favorite memory was when she told me I had a "Coming appetite." I would declare I wasn't hungry. The more I ate, the hungrier I became. Must confess that I still have that coming appetite.

Follow Others: Aging Wisdom from Beatitudes, Nature, Kinfolk

Like Mother, Like Son. Recently many of us cousins attended the funeral of our Uncle Jesse. He passed away at 89 and the funeral remembrances honored him as a loving parent. Although never a father himself, he helped raise and inspire nine young men—six plus one girl as a step dad, also his own three younger brothers 14, 12, and 11 when they lost their dad and Jesse was 18.

Turns out that both Flora and son Jesse had each raised ten children, with so much love and skill that they will be long remembered and are not replaceable.

"A good life gets passed on to the grandchildren." Proverbs 13:22, the Message

Personality Types or Temperaments. God must like diversity, because even to Hippocrates, a Greek philosopher, it was obvious that there were at least four different temperaments, each with a recognizable (predictable) abundance of personality traits. Because the differences were thought to stem from the four bodily fluid types, the names he chose were related to what was thought to exist in human bodies. The theory of temperaments fell out of favor until the 1970s. That's when Christian author, Tim LaHaye reintroduced and expanded upon the temperament types in many books.

Although each person has a dominant and subsidiary temperament, definitions given below are for dominant traits only:

Melancholic—If it can be over-thought and worried about a Melancholic is just the temperament to do it. Detail-oriented, with a love to research and organize data, they often work as engineers or in other technical jobs. The melancholic child can get straight As in school, except in typing and drivers education.

Follow Others: Aging Wisdom from Beatitudes, Nature, Kinfolk

Sanguine—Why worry or study when you can party, talk and otherwise enjoy life with other people? That is the Sanguine's philosophy. They are excellent at sales or care/service jobs. The sanguine child will want to sleep with a pet.

Choleric—The true leader, they thrive on decisions and are intuitive planners. What they recommend is what everyone else should do or say. The Choleric child will be the leader of his/her siblings no matter what rank they hold in the birth order (first born, middle child, baby, only child). To learn more about birth order and personalities, read The Birth Order Book by Dr. Kevin Leman.

Phlegmatic—This temperament knows how to be content and patient. They only need others to leave them in peace and not mess with their possessions. Faithful and dependable, they perform many functions in the financial, manufacturing and service industries. The Phlegmatic child may be overweight by the age of five.

Financial Flaws and Strengths by Temperaments. We human beings are not good at making judgments about ourselves. In fact we are apt to accept blame or take credit for things we may not have done alone. I found learning about personalities helped me better accept the way I am, while understanding where I need to ask for help to improve. Finances is one of those areas of improvement needed for me.

Sanguine—Anyone who has this personality type as their primary trait will be generous to a fault. Reining in the desire for new, pretty or more things will early on be a difficult task, with restraint coming from a secondary trait or the traits of a life partner. This type may mourn the loss of funding after retirement and as generous family and friends pass away.

Choleric—If a choleric can stay out of business debt and humbly involve their mate in decisions, they will prosper and achieve their

Follow Others: Aging Wisdom from Beatitudes, Nature, Kinfolk

lifetime goals. The choleric needs to learn to show and receive love. This type will mourn the loss of supporter or help meet.

Melancholic—This personality type is most guilty of expecting perfection of themselves and others. They do not take the blame for overstepping their income. This type will mourn the loss of friends who admired their intelligence and accepted their failings.

Phlegmatic—This type loves to save and rarely spends money. They may own several income producing properties and drive an older model vehicle. They need to practice generosity and put plans in action. They may mourn the loss of up-lifters.

Retirement by the Temperaments. There is no one-way people act regarding retirement. My spouse just turned 66 and became eligible to retire. He considers this an advantage due to a down economy where youth are more often hired. I see it as an advantage to do consulting work, with many life-time workers leaving the market. There is always a need for those who have answers and ability. Below are some possible responses to retirement based on temperaments:

Sanguines—miss being around people. They should get a pet, though they most likely already have one. They can become the perfect volunteers with their caring empathetic personality.

Cholerics—miss the decision making and being in control of major projects. First place to start is redoing their own home and/or moving as they always meant to do. They can start a consulting business with its combination of responsibility and free time; they need to balance these wisely to enjoy senior life.

Melancholics—consume much of their free time imagining the worst-case health scenarios, unless they have already realized worry is like sitting in a rocking chair—it goes nowhere. With their talent they can write a book/memoir, offer to mentor a young person or edit books for author wannabes.

Follow Others: Aging Wisdom from Beatitudes, Nature, Kinfolk

Phlegmatics—tempted to procrastinate on dealing with health issues, especially without company paid insurance. Many will have false teeth due to liking sweets and having put off dentist work in youth. They should make sure they have good insurance, with a reasonable deductible, such as one of the Medicare-related plans offered by insurance companies. Hobbies, such as coin collecting, allow one to start small and invest at the same time. See the chapter on Adventure.

Ways to Earn Money Post Retirement. The source of our primary earnings will come as a result of our primary personality temperament. However, when it comes time to earn extra spending money after retirement, or for a quick income earning job, we should look for sources based on our second temperament.

Sanguines—can flash a smile at a customer better than any other personality type. Small businesses like a deli, 7-11, or grocery store would love your part-time help as a cashier or customer service rep.

Cholerics—should invest in purchasing the tools of their primary trade or for a nascent hobby/calling: software, drill press, advanced degree. Consultant pay is extremely lucrative even when pursued part-time. Christian charities could use your leadership expertise.

Melancholics—can share talents for writing, graphic art and teaching. Write a book or create an online course, then master online marketing. Volunteer as a missionary helper for room and board.

Phlegmatics—consider managing money earned and saved in their lifetime as a second job; therefore don't ask them for a loan. However, sharing financial advice is the best legacy a phlegmatic can leave behind. And they can always work in a grocery store if they want to be out among people.

Follow Others: Aging Wisdom from Beatitudes, Nature, Kinfolk

End Point: Actions follow thoughts. To break a negative cycle refuse to do the action. Rather try prayer that God change your view. Then you can say, "My God supplies all my needs according to his riches in glory..", paraphrase of Philippians 4:19

Prayer Point: And as you would that men should do to you, do ye also to them likewise. Luke 6:31

Follow Others: Aging Wisdom from Beatitudes, Nature, Kinfolk

Follow Others: Aging Wisdom from Beatitudes, Nature, Kinfolk

Beatitude: God will wipe away every tear from their eyes, and death shall be no more neither shall there be anguish—sorrow and mourning—nor grief nor pain any more: for the old conditions and former order of things have passed away. Revelation 21:4 Amplified

Chapter 14—Push To the Top

Consider this: Beatitudes are the Psalms summarized; the Epistles are the Beatitudes applied.

This chapter of Follow Others focuses on working out the plan for the remainder of our years.

There is no harder experience than to insist that a relative with Alzheimer's disease must no longer drive. We pulled my mother-in-law's license when she was in her eighties. She knocked over a mail box on the side of a road driving home from her weekly bowling. We sold her car and the nastiness began. She would look up from a book or newspaper and condemn us for selling the car. This happened repeatedly, almost as long as she was able to remain in the house before going to a nursing home. When we left her in a room at the home, she threatened to walk to her house because she knew where she was—several miles away on a major route atop a local mountain. Fortunately, she never tried, finally forgetting her reason for being disgruntled.

Meet Again at the Top. By the time we are aged, we have said goodbye to many dear folk, some like those you have read my tales of remembrance in this book. How much more difficult it is to say a final goodbye to our own loved ones—parents, spouse and even children? Jesus offered the hope that we would see them once again in a place referred to as heaven.

Follow Others: Aging Wisdom from Beatitudes, Nature, Kinfolk

Decisions at Base Camp:

Burial or Cremation; see Upper Taker or Undertaker section.

Marry Again or Stay Single; see Single Aging Roundup.

Move or not; see Next move, New Mountain section.

Upper Taker or Undertaker. I remember one thing my Uncle Ed preached about aging. He would insist to his congregation of older folk "We are not looking for the undertaker, but for the upper-taker." He may have referred to verses in the book of Revelation as preached on by Charles H. Spurgeon in the below sermon.

After these things I looked, and behold, a door standing open in heaven. And the first voice which I heard was like a trumpet speaking with me, saying, "Come up here, and I will show you things which must take place after this." Immediately I was in the Spirit; and behold, a throne set in heaven, and One sat on the throne. Revelations 4: 1-2 (NKJ)

CH Spurgeon, Sermon. I was told of a poor peasant in the mountains who, month after month, year after year, through a long period of declining life, opened his casement every morning, as soon as he awoke, and looked toward the east to see if Jesus Christ was coming. He had not calculated the date of Christ's coming, or he would not have needed to look at all. He was ready for Christ's coming, or he would not have been in such a hurry to seek him. He was willing for Christ's coming, or he would rather have looked another way. He loved, or Christ would not have been the first thought of the morning. His Master did not come, but eventually a messenger did, to fetch the ready one home. The same preparation sufficed for both; his longing soul was satisfied with either. Often the child of God awakes in the morning, weary and encumbered with troubled thoughts, and his Father's secret presence comes to mind. He looks up (if not out) to feel (if not to see)

Follow Others: Aging Wisdom from Beatitudes, Nature, Kinfolk

the glories of that last morning when the trumpet shall sound and the dead shall arise indestructible--no weary limbs to bear the spirit down; no feverish dreams to haunt the vision; no dark forecasting of the day's events, no returning memory of the grief of yesterday.

Burial Expenses. When my Uncle Ed passed away we learned one fact about burial expenses. It doesn't matter where you hold the funeral, the undertaker charges for his services. That is why It is important to get a written explanation of all services to be provided and an itemized list of the costs. Expect, at this time, the cost to be a minimum of $8000 for the funeral and burial expenses.

Some insurance plans can help with these costs by a monthly premium charge paid ahead of time. They often advertise their plans/costs on national afternoon TV.

My Uncle and his wife both died this past winter in Vermont, each a month or so apart. Their children opted for a single burial service in the spring so they could be interred together. A heart-warming ending to a long love story.

Cremation or Plot. Does your family have any unused spots in their burial plot? This option is worth checking into as plots in any cemetery are not cheap. My ex-husband will be buried next to his bachelor uncles; there was one spot never used by the family. Ashes in a cremation urn can be buried, too.

To research burial spots, you can search a registry like Ancestry. Or search online in old township records for where relatives may be buried. You'll learn a lot about your ancestors, regardless of whether or not you find an open plot.

Follow Others: Aging Wisdom from Beatitudes, Nature, Kinfolk

Some folk may wish to be cremated. Pros and cons, beside personal preference.

Pros for Cremation: Accident that caused disfigurement; Death outside the state where burial is to be made. This cuts embalming and transportation costs.; Time considerations, like death in winter that postpones burial.

Cons for Cremation: Some churches do not approve; Some wish to be buried as were their relatives; Costs are not typically lower, either for burial or cremation.

Life Changes. As you become aware of health issues, refer to the chapters 8-9 in this book. I have included many natural and simple heath tips for you to try. And most are inexpensive, from herbs to ointments. The best remedy is to get up and get moving. Here's some advice about exercise—even young athletes experience pain that limits them from doing all they want to. What they do differently than aging folk, is they don't blow it all out of proportion. They understand that a minor back injury, like a pulled muscle, will heal itself in a week. The biggest problem for the athlete will be sitting still until it heals and they get back moving.

Pain Management. Beside the following section on pain management, read the Therapy and Therapists section in chapter 12.

Pain management is an upcoming medical field as Opioid addiction becomes responsible for making drug addicts of those who deal with pain and subsequently our children. Nowadays, many seniors are becoming more knowledgeable about how to use natural ingredients, like herbs and homeopathy, to relieve ongoing pain.

Follow Others: Aging Wisdom from Beatitudes, Nature, Kinfolk

Refer to earlier sections that provide advice on using these ingredients for specific issues to help manage temporary pain. Also see the discussion of Ointments and Treatments along with Homeopathy Basics in Chapter 12.

Drugs and Side Effects—Opioid Addiction. There was a time when doctors freely prescribed opioid medication for nagging pan. They still prescribe it after surgery; I have a bottle of Percocet sitting in my bathroom cabinet left from my shoulder surgery a past April. I took one dose to sleep the first night home from the hospital.

I am so thankful that I could never handle prescription medicines well. This is why I discovered early on homeopathic healing remedies, like Arnica Montana mentioned earlier. So sad that many people have resorted to taking doctor prescriptions long enough to become addicted.

Steroids Replacing Antibiotics. Now that antibiotics have been prescribed for so many infections, bacteria have become resistant to some of these life-saving medicines. Doctors are instead prescribing steroids to pump up a person's immune system for anything they consider viral, like upper respiratory colds and sinus infections.

Steroids too have negative effects such as:

Taking them too frequently can cause early-onset cataracts.

They can make a mild-mannered woman act like an aggressive male (just saying).

They can cause problems with holding fluids and in the digestive system.

Over the Counter (OTC) products. Now doctors are advising not to take aspirin as prevention against heart attacks. I just realized that ibuprofen raises my blood pressure. Cough medicines can prolong a cough. Fortunately, I have discovered homeopathic remedies which can give me the desired results. Other seniors use aromatherapy as a safe option.

Follow Others: Aging Wisdom from Beatitudes, Nature, Kinfolk

CDB products. Medicinal marijuana is legal in all states, so can be found for sale as CBD oil in any health food store. Medicinal marijuana does not have hallucinogenic ingredients.

Possible side effects of CBD oil:

Sleepiness; take in smaller doses.

Stomach issues similar to those caused by marijuana, which are relieved by taking a hot bath or shower.

Herbal Healers. Seniors are savvy shoppers of natural pain remedies. I will mention only a few herbs that are well-known for reducing pain due to inflammation. Since I have little personal experience, I will invite my readers to share your stories with other readers on my blog at http://donnaaford.com.

Turmeric Curcumin. This antioxidant component of the herb, turmeric, is touted as a destroyer of free radicals which contribute to the aging process. Check that any Turmeric herbal preparation delivers a standardized amount of curcumin. Prolonged use can cause gall bladder response. Curcumin is said to:

Support joints. My daughter takes it to relieve knee pain from a fall while a teen.

Reduce the effects of aging on skin, hair and body.

Enhance immune system. I now sprinkle it instead whenever salt is called for in a recipe.

Improve digestion. Shares this ability with its botanical relative ginger root.

Follow Others: Aging Wisdom from Beatitudes, Nature, Kinfolk

Capsicum/Capsaicin. This component of chili peppers is best known as the chemical used in pepper spray. In its less potent forms it can be used to treat a multitude of ailments such as:

Fevers

Congestion due to colds and sinus

Topical rub on for muscle and joint pain, including arthritis

Skin and nerve pain such as shingles

More recently, it is touted for losing weight. Interestingly, since I reached my seventies, I enjoying spicier menu items. I remember my mother eagerly eating hot cherry peppers when she was about this age. Our bodies know what works for us.

Ginger. During my hip injury and healing time, I used an ointment that contains ginger. It reduces inflammation if rubbed on the painful area. Helps with colds.

Homeopathic Healing. Arnicare is a group of products whose major homeopathic ingredient is Arnica Montana. Arnicare products are distributed in gel or cream forms for surface application to injured muscles.

Other homeopathic healers like T-relief (formerly Traumeel) are in tablet format to be taken orally. T-relief is a combination of remedies that can be taken orally whenever a topical application would not suit the injury, or rubbed on as a cream. This includes a portion of Arnica as well. I first ran across this product when I partially injured the rotator cuff of my left shoulder from helping my spouse sheetrock the garage. I first tried acupuncture treatments, then physical therapy but nothing relieved the discomfort of lifting my arm up to get dressed. On my last visit to the acupuncturist she handed me a bottle of Traumeel that a salesperson had left with her. This is hard to belief, but within a few short days my left shoulder began to heal and has never bothered since.

Arnica Montana is a homeopathic remedy made from a mountain daisy that grows in Montana which is known for its healing properties. As opposed to pain medicines, Arnica helps heal injured areas, and thus relieves the pain of healing. A few people may be allergic to Arnica, since it is derived from an herb.

Take Arnica pellets from Boiron: 30c is the best dosage for an acute pain or recent injury, such as aches from falling off your bicycle or another type accident. Take orally whenever pain from healing is felt; After a surgery, take Arnica Montana 200c to help wean yourself off of pain medication as soon as possible.

Give Up Independence

"..forgetting those things which are behind, and reaching for those before, I press toward the mark for the prize of the high calling of God.."Philippians 3:13, 14

Personal independence is nearly our final battle. No one wants to depend on others, since the garden of Eden story proves that even our teammate's help can't always be trusted.

Not Able to Drive. I sincerely hope that none of my readers have had to make this change from driver to passive passenger, which most seniors consider one of the worst changes. When you can no longer drive, for whatever reason, you must depend on others, taxis or public transportation to go shopping, doctor appointments, anywhere. I'm too much an independent New Englander to wish that on anyone. After

Follow Others: Aging Wisdom from Beatitudes, Nature, Kinfolk

seventy-five, my state requires an eye exam before renewal. Check your state's requirements.

Aunt Who Hit Trooper's Car. My spouse's aunt drove a large station wagon well into her eighties. One day she ran into a State Trooper vehicle at an intersection. Aware of the consequences since she had cataracts, she did not resist her lost license. The car was promptly bought by her daughter and driven to another state.

Uber and Lyft. With these recent companies able to provide rides at all hours of the day, getting around without a car/license is somewhat easier. Of course, one must always be careful about safety when using an unknown service. Contact for details: www.uber.com or www.lyft.com

From Car to Cane and Walker. More limiting is when the person requires a cane or walker to get around in their home. The one bright spot: family members who become chauffeurs get to utilize the state-issued handicapped parking sticker.

Pets. And of course, the ultimate giving up of independence is to move out of one's own home. If you have pets, unfortunately they will need to find a new home as well. You could still "adopt" a pet owned by someone else. Nursing homes often have a resident pet. Or visit a dog walk area and make friends with some owners.

Uncle Ed – Looking for Uppertaker (his story continued from Chapter 2). I remember one thing Uncle Ed preached about aging. He would insist to his congregation of older folk "We are not looking for the undertaker, but for the upper-taker." He referred to the Bible's description of a future date when Jesus will return and catch his living church up into the air to be forever with him.

Follow Others: Aging Wisdom from Beatitudes, Nature, Kinfolk

"We shall not all sleep, but we shall all be changed, In a moment in a twinkling of the eye...this mortal must put on immortality." I Corinthians 15:51-53

The undertaker unfortunately won in Hardwick, as Uncle Ed and most of his congregation have passed before that promised day. The Parkinson's disease forced him quit his job as night watchmen at a hospital a half-hour drive from home. I road with him once, me praying as we careened around some of those corners. He gave up his long fight in a nursing home two weeks after losing a leg to amputation. I never even made it there for a visit, but my husband did. Contemplating a future of sitting in a wheel chair must have been anathema to this athletic person even in his 80s.

I still can't make any plans about a purchasing a burial plot or insurance without hearing his confident voice declare with hope and courage, "We are not looking for the undertaker.."

Single-ager Roundup. Early on in writing this book, I received a suggestion that one class of seniors has been neglected in most books on Aging—the single seniors group. The special needs of singles was mentioned to me during a recent discussion with a church member whose ministry is among their aging congregation.

Aging can be difficult enough within an immediate support system. Some spouses pass away within hours of each other but not always. How do newly-single people fare when they begin to experience the limitations associated with aging? Missing companionship may be their most trying obstacle to resuming life as usual. Consider including these people in church gatherings.

Female singles might appreciate help with caring for cars and doing taxes. They may appreciate help to sell a home or downsize household items.

Follow Others: Aging Wisdom from Beatitudes, Nature, Kinfolk

Male singles may need instruction in doing simple tasks, such as how to wash clothes, cook simple meals and run washer/dryer. When I fell and broke my femur, my spouse helped by learning how to wash clothes and dishes. Widowers also may need advice on how to meet available women of suitable age.

Most singles would appreciate help with having to make decisions alone, unless they have friends, children or church family they can trust. Even if you don't see how you could offer advice, just being a good listener is the best help. I need to talk out important decisions. Once when all my support people were unavailable and I needed to make a significant decision, I ended up talking to the person in my apartment building's sales office. Of course she couldn't advise, but I with her listening was able to recognize the direction best suited for me.

"Trust in the Lord with all [your] heart; and lean not unto [your] own understanding. In all [your] ways acknowledge him, and he shall direct [your] paths," Proverbs 3:5, 6 KJV, modified

Next Move, New Mountain. "In my Father's house are many mansions: if it were not so, I would have told you. I go to prepare a place for you..that where I am, there you may be also." John 14:2-3

I read a book written by the wife of a service man. Bekah DiFelice had moved with her brand-new husband and then repeatedly to other places he was stationed. I bought the book to give to my grandson's wife since he is in the Coast Guard and is now stationed in Alaska.

However, some of the author's comments struck home for anyone who must move reluctantly. Here are a few of her words of wisdom regarding moves.

Home doesn't begin or end with a mailing address or change in surname.

Follow Others: Aging Wisdom from Beatitudes, Nature, Kinfolk

Good news. We never arrive to empty rooms empty handed.

Faith is a bridge between places.

"None are so old as those who have outlived enthusiasm." Henry David Thoreau who lived in a one room cabin at Walden Pond

I love the idea of owning less stuff and seeing less clutter everyday as I walk through the ten rooms of our Greek-revival farm house. However, I know where this topic is going. What I now perceive as freedom must one day become limitations.

When you must make three lists—what to keep, what to give away and what to trash—consider this with an upbeat frame of mind. Here are some positives:

Travel—If you opt for a travel home, you can visit relatives frequently and see places you've only read about. Get a copy of the book 50 States 5000 Ideas, published by National Geographic, and make plans for a travel trip or many; Join the Road Scholars tours; search online for details.

New Home—A smaller home or apartment will cost less to rent/own and less to heat. It also means less time spent dusting/cleaning; Two-story homes are difficult for those who have been injured or suffer from arthritis. Sell the house or install a stair lift. Buy two vacuum cleaners, one for each floor.

Retirement home—Do you already own the perfect spot in a lovely state? Wow, I wish I were you and hope it's a log cabin in the mountains. Still you will need to make plans to visit family and friends in the old neighborhood at least once or twice a year. Although Zoom phone calls can make it seem like you never moved away.

Follow Others: Aging Wisdom from Beatitudes, Nature, Kinfolk

Residence home—What can you take? Assisted living spaces include a kitchen, bedroom and sitting area. The nursing homes typically require you to share a room with some other patient. Single rooms are too expensive to afford on Social Security payments. I don't know about you, but I haven't shared a room with anyone I didn't know since college days. Not sure how that would go, but my children and their spouses have all informed me I can't move in with them. I'm going to agree about that—for now anyways.

Hire a professional. Or arrange for relatives to share the care of an aged individual. Problems to consider:

Sleepless nights

Dealing with confusion from Dementia and Alzheimer's

Patience and good humor required by caregiver

Physical strength to lift or move patient

Hospice—is the final destination for those dealing with debilitating health issues, including cancer, heart and liver failure and advanced brain diseases. The expected time to spend in hospice is two weeks. Professional administration of drugs to cover pain result in an early demise. My mother opted at 83 not to have abdominal surgery for a twisted bowel resection. An opiate was administered in increasing doses until she passed away. Any relative who experiences hospice knows this is not an easy decision.

More about Temporary Homes. With the aging of the baby boomers, an entire home care/health care industry has come into being. I asked my sister who worked in this industry what advice she could give for those making decisions. She recommended a website called, A Place for

Follow Others: Aging Wisdom from Beatitudes, Nature, Kinfolk

Mom. The website explains the various types of care offered. The right choice will depend on these things: the physical and emotional needs of the client, whether they can drive and how much the options cost. The site lists a few places to look for funding, including Veterans Aid and Assistance and Medicaid. There are some sources for low-cost loans against your present home. Contact an Elder Care Attorney for help. Choosing a Christian Care Community may best suit your aging relative; call 888-901-0627 to learn about options near your home. You will find their website at: www.aPlaceForMom.com.

Making this important next-step decision, the site suggests a four-step process:

Evaluate facilities in your area

Schedule a tour earlier than later. Make this scheduled visit at meal time so your loved one can meet the residents

Pop in at some other time of day for a second visit.

Check that the seniors and staff seem happy. Trust your gut feelings.

Last Memories

Aunt Letha's Story. You met my Great Aunt Letha earlier in this book. She and her husband Val cut their own firewood, made maple syrup from their sap trees and was independent up until the time she had to leave their home high on a Vermont hillside. One of Val's nephews had looked in on her since her husband passed away. He brought her down off the hillside one last time to live in her relative's home. I drove over to visit her there once; they had prepared her a separate room about the size at any nursing home. They cared for her lovingly, but too soon I learned of her passing. Some people are too independent to last long even in the comfort of a relative's home. Good bye, Aunt Letha.

Follow Others: Aging Wisdom from Beatitudes, Nature, Kinfolk

Grandma Ford – Alzheimer's Couldn't Steal Hope. At first, my mother-in-law could not remember days of the week. Then we observed that she did not recognize her own relatives at a funeral. When we discovered that she cooked meatloaf most days for supper, her son moved in with her. Eventually she failed until she could not reopen the unlocked front door after walking outside in the rain. This was the point at which we realized she needed round-the-clock care.

When she first moved into the nursing home she got very angry. Alzheimer patients are happier to be in familiar surroundings. Soon it became familiar too, or else she forgot why she had been angry. About six months later, she celebrated her 91st birthday. When I visited, I helped her look through the stack of cards received. She had always remembered others and this last time of her life they remembered her. I commented out loud that many people loved her, along with us. Then I added that God loved her, too. Her reply was a almost a question: I hope He does. Her Methodist minister had visited her recently and she may have been considering this concept. I assured her that God did indeed love her. That was our last conversation, which proves that the disease can not steal all our thoughts.

Interesting that she who lived with a strong-willed father and then husband, wondered if she had done enough to please God. If you knew her, you would understand how this dear, sweet woman, like a second mother to me since fifteen, always perfectly fit her name: Grace.

For details about this disease see the Alzheimer's /Dementia section Chapter 6.

Follow Others: Aging Wisdom from Beatitudes, Nature, Kinfolk

End Point: What will matter most at the end of life are: People we've loved and served; Memories of those who loved us; Our relationship with God.

Prayer Point: And even to your old age I am he; and even to [grey] hairs will I carry you... Isaiah 46:4a

Follow Others: Aging Wisdom from Beatitudes, Nature, Kinfolk

Afterword, About

Consider this: "Tough choices ahead." I predicted several times in this book that there are two places/times in our later years we will have to re-evaluate the plan for aging. The first comes when we reach our fifties and AARP sends their ubiquitous magazine. How did they find us so soon?

The second time comes when our level of living is less than satisfactory, perhaps in the late 70s or 80s. We have less mobility, less income, have lost a partner, must move out of our home, etc. In this day and age, many will not have to make this evaluation until well past their seventies. Regardless of when, there will be tough choices ahead. Make these choices we must, always considering that we may live well into our nineties—like my kinfolk.

"Two Paths..I Took the Road Less Travelled". As we make our final plans, we have two options. We can decide, like an 80+ neighbor did recently when diagnosed with returning pancreatic cancer, that everything wrong with her made life unbearable.

Or we can weather on regardless of the struggles ahead for the sake of those we care for and about—like when we recently climbed a mountain in NH to look for semi-precious gems. I slowed down our progress with many stops for water and energy bar snacks, but we finally made it together to our destination. Either path is honorable!

Do I really want to live to be 100? What does my choice depend on? Some questions to ask yourself:

Quality of life? Health and stamina; Finances

Support of friends/family; what if they die younger?

Follow Others: Aging Wisdom from Beatitudes, Nature, Kinfolk

Last Goodbyes. Almost everyone has a story to tell of some miraculous or unexplained happening when saying final goodbyes to a loved one. Like Billy Graham's grandma, some dying sit bolt upright in bed and talk to a deceased love one. Others are clearly seeing people or beings beyond this world, as indicated by the eye movements of a friend's mother. Such stories are not surprising when our loved ones are close to crossing over the line between two existences. Our love for them permits us a brief peak behind that curtain.

Who is with the dying person when they draw their final breath? My mother lived as long as we four daughters were in the room talking about her. When we all left, she died in the presence of my brother instead. Another friend was sad that she hadn't been there when her father died. I commented that he might not have passed away with her in the room. The dying absolutely do know who is in the room with them.

Premonitions. One person told that she would die on the 18th of the month; another that he would die at 8 o'clock. They were each right. I felt certain that my father would be the first of my close family to pass away and at 72 he was. For the first time in 18 years, I heard my father's voice just before my mother died. Clear as day I heard in my head him gruffly speak my name, as he often did when he wanted my attention. It seemed he was telling me to let her go without insisting she have the surgery that could have spared her life.

Apostle Paul's Near Death Experience (NDE). Paul told the Christian believers in Corinth that he would not boast about himself. Instead he mentioned a man "in the body or out of it, I cannot tell" who was caught up to the Heavens and witnessed glories. At various cities where he preached, Paul was beaten and stoned; he was also adrift on the seas. We do not know the exact incident that resulted in his NDE, but the

Follow Others: Aging Wisdom from Beatitudes, Nature, Kinfolk

recount of it in II Corinthians 11: 23-25 and 12: 1-5, 11 is worth reading. You will notice he juxtaposes the words "glory" and 'weak" seven times each.

Final Visit with the Kinfolk. VT Fatherland and Bert G

Technically, I was the last female child raised by my mom's father. I was born into his household when my mother came home to stay during World War II. My one distant memory is of his bald head highlighted in the morning sun that came through the window as he sat at the kitchen table. My playpen shared the same room, both of us confined—him by poor health and me by wooden playpen bars. The next memory I have was after my dad returned from the war and we had moved out-of-state. Grandpa's mind was failing fast (hardening of the arteries they called dementia in 1948) and his family all came to visit. A hired photographer captured us gathered around the couch in his living room. That was the last picture taken with him. But I had "forgotten" Grandpa long before that day; as a five year old the picture shows me snuggled with my grandma instead. A child does not understand when a grandparent no longer acknowledges them.

When I took up poetry writing in college, I researched Grandpa's history. Scottish relatives arrived on the Mayflower. The family of stone masons would move to Barre, VT, near the famous rock quarries. Grandpa worked in one of the sheds near Barre as a lumper, moving slabs of granite between cutting stations to where carvers would shape and embellish into grave stones. In the 1930s, many shed workers went on strike. They demanded vacuum systems installed to remove the stone dust polluting the air which caused deaths of industry workers from lung disease, Silicosis. My grandpa was expected to strike too, but he refused to take food and money from the organizers. Even with a big family to feed, he didn't believe it right to accept payment for doing

Follow Others: Aging Wisdom from Beatitudes, Nature, Kinfolk

nothing. Sometimes I struggle mentally with collecting Social Security. I must have inherited a bit of his Vermont independent streak!

It is interesting to note that his sons all lived to be older than he was at death, even though most of them worked in granite sheds, too. Apparently, ventilation of the work areas really did lengthen many lives.

Which Path Are You On?

A Crutch? Certain people claim that religion is one of those crutches we grab when we are desperate. I might point out, though, that if the religious "crutch" didn't work in this age of online shopping, we'd quickly order a new four-footed cane or transport chair from Amazon. The fact that last minute conversions hold up over time proves them to be real, sincere.

Do you hope or do you know? I wanted to see signs or wonders before I believed what the Bible claimed about Jesus being the Son of God. I preferred to create my own kingdom with rules of my own choosing—one where things were always fair according to my standards. It took a miscarriage that ended my second pregnancy to convince me that I should reconsider accepting Jesus' offer of a new kingdom.

Join in Jesus' Kingdom. Once I decided to let God rule the universe, not me, an amazing peace came over my life. This peace has lasted for fifty years now. I recommend that you research the kingdom blessings promised by the Beatitudes in chapters 2-5. May you know this peace for yourself.

Follow Others: Aging Wisdom from Beatitudes, Nature, Kinfolk

End Point: I would love to hear that something you learned within this book has been of help to you. Please contact me at: author@donnaaford.com

Prayer Point: "To laugh often and much; to win the respect of intelligent people and the affection of children..to leave the world a better place..to know even one life has breathed easier because you have lived. This is to have succeeded." Ralph Waldo Emerson

About

Photos. All photos of the Grand Teton mountain trails were taken by the author on a hike near Jackson Hole, Wyoming in 2003. The photograph of Corliss kinfolk was taken by an attendee of the 1965 Corliss reunion held in Vermont. They were all in their seventies at the time.

Resources. Refer to that section at the end of the book to see titles and dates of all the nutritional books that form the basis of the author's education on healthy aging. She still owns many of the original books where she learned about Health.

Author Website: http://donnaaford.com

Biographies for Young Adults by the Author

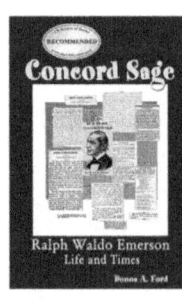 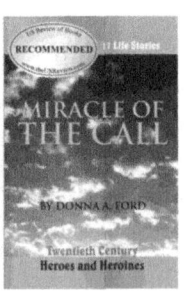

Concord Sage: Ralph Waldo Emerson Life and Times, published through Inspiring Voices, May 2015; Recommended by the US Review of Books; Available at Amazon in kindle or paper back.

Miracle of the Call: Twentieth Century Heroes and Heroines, published through Westbow Press, December 2015; Recommended by the US Review of Books; The Eric Hoffer Award Winner, Honorable Mention 2017; Available at Amazon in kindle, paper back or hardcover.

Appendix A—Personal Health Defense

In case someone wonders, here is how I use herbs and homeopathy to defend myself from colds and flu prevalent in winter time. For better results, space out the time between taking each homeopathic remedy. [Note that because of high blood pressure, I should not use standard OTC cold products. Also, note that the herbs I choose work well for blood type A.]

Use in Advance of Colds:

A&D capsules or cod liver oil capsules—higher potencies in cold weather; Reduce amount of A taken in warm weather to avoid leg pains

Echinacea 2x day; stop after 2 weeks—(all members of the house if any family member has a cold); Essential for Blood Type A

Homeopathic—*Natrum Muriaticum (stress); *Gelsenium (travelling or stage fright)

Take at Start of Colds/Flu:

Chewable zinc tablets (twice a day)

Echinacea (2 to 3 times per day)—Works best for Blood Type A

Fiber or mild laxative

OTC product for allergy relief (once a day) Claritin—(better than Zertek for long lasting issue); Allergy nasal spray

Follow Others: Aging Wisdom from Beatitudes, Nature, Kinfolk

Homeopathic—*Gelsenium (flu with chills); *Hepar sulphuris calcareum (sore throat especially if exposure to strep); *Belladonna (fever with red cheeks);*Nux Vomica (stomach and diarrhea);*Euphrasia (pink eye);*Oscillococcium (flu; take one whole tube)

Hand reflexology for adrenal gland stimulation—Rub points in palm: middle of palm; under base of thumb and thumb pad; Squeeze both sides at base of wrist; lightly rub back of hand

Colds that Don't Respond to Above:

Raw garlic (natural antibiotic)—Cut into tiny pieces and swallow 1 tsp 3x a day

Ashwagandha (for those with low resistance)—Works best for Blood Type A

Acupuncture treatment

OTC products—nasal decongestion and cough (check if safe for those with high blood pressure); Antibiotic from doctor

Homeopathic—*Kali Bichromium (laryngitis without cough; stringy phlegm; bronchitis); *Kali Muriaticum (left ear stuffed up); *Pulsitilla (thick green phlegm); *Rumex (dry cough with fever); *Spongia tosta (cough with wheezing; laryngitis with cough)

Aromatherapy–peppermint oil

Hand reflexology for sinus stimulation—Sinus pressure points are at the base of each fingernail on the pad side of the finger; also between the web of pointer and ring fingers. Apply pressure by digging a fingernail or squeezing each pressure point. You should feel pressure relief and flowing of nasal fluid out of sinus.

Follow Others: Aging Wisdom from Beatitudes, Nature, Kinfolk

Stressful Situations:

Hand reflexology for Relaxation–Intertwine and squeeze fingers firmly; hold until calm

Aromatherapy–lavender, peppermint oil

Homeopathic—Ignatia Amara* (restlessness during sleep hours due to thinking) or (losses) (terrifying experiences); Gelsemium Sempervirens* (travel or speaking events)

*All homeopathic Boiron remedies used for acute (not longstanding) scenarios are 30c potency; dissolve 3 pills in mouth 2 or 3 times per day, every hour if very ill. Try another remedy if no improvement noticed shortly. I highly recommend purchasing a homeopathic reference book. See Resources.

Follow Others: Aging Wisdom from Beatitudes, Nature, Kinfolk

Resources

Health/healing:

Adelle Davis, Let's Get Well, Harcourt, Brace & World, 1965

Joyce Gardner Prensky/ Joy Garner, Healing Yourself, 6th addition, self-printed, 1966-1967; The New Healing Yourself: Natural Remedies for Adults and Children, The Crossing Press, 1989

Dr. Carl C. Pfeiffer, Zinc and Other Micro-Nutrients, Keats Publishing, 1978

Bernard Jensen, D.C, Nutritionist, Iridology Simplified, And Introduction to the Sciences of Iridology and its Relation to Nutrition, Iridologists International, 1980

John Parks Trowbridge, MD/Morton Walker, D.P.M.,The Yeast Syndrome: How to Help Your Doctor Identify and Treat the Real Cause of Your Yeast-related Illness, Bantam Books, 1986

Stephen T. Sinatra, MD/Jan Sinatra, RN, MSN/Roberta Jo Lieberman,Heart Sense for Women, Your Plan for Natural Prevention and Treatment, Penguin Group, 2001

Dr. Andrew Lockie, The Family Guide To Homeopathy: Symptoms and Natural Solutions, Fireside Simon & Schuster,1989

Stephen Cummings, MD/Dana Ullman, MPH, Everybody's Guide to Homeopathic Medicines: Taking Care of Yourself and Your Family with Safe and Effective Remedies, Jeremy P. Tracher/Perigee Books, 1991

Follow Others: Aging Wisdom from Beatitudes, Nature, Kinfolk

Diet/nutrition:

Jean Hewitt, The New York Times Natural Food Cookbook, Times Books, 1971

Frances Moore Lappe, Diet for a Small Planet, Ballatine books, 1971

Ellen Buchmen Ewald, Recipes for a Small Planet, Ballatine books, 1977; "Started a revolution in the way Americans eat."

Dr. Peter J. D'Adamo/Catherine Whitney, Eat Right For Your Type: Complete Blood Type Encyclopedia, Riverhead Books/Penguin Putnam, 2002

Casey Kellar and Nicole Kellar-Munoz, Quick-Fix Healthy Mix: 225 Health and Affordable Mix Recipes to Stock Your Kitchen, Krause Publications, 2009

Rick Warren/Daniel Amen/Mark Hyman, The Daniel Plan: 40 Days to a Healthier Life, Zondervan, 2013

William Davis, MD, Wheat Belly: Lose the Wheat, Lose the Weight, and Find Your Path Back to Health, Rodale, 2013

Steven R. Gundry, MD, The Longevity Paradox, How to Die Young at a Ripe Old Age, Harper Wave, 2019

Exercise/massage:

Bonnie Prudden, Pain Erasure: The Bonnie Prudden Way, Ballantine, 1980; newer releases available

Mildred Carter/Tammy Weber, Hand Reflexology: Key to Perfect Health, Revised & Expanded, Prentice Hall, 2000 (had earlier version)

Follow Others: Aging Wisdom from Beatitudes, Nature, Kinfolk

Devaki Berkson, The Foot Book; Haling the Body Through Reflexology, Harper Perennial, 1992

Asa Hershoff, ND, DC, Homeopathy for Musculoskeletal Healing, North Atlantic Books, 1996

Christine Ann Kent, Save Your Hips: Heal Hip Pain Naturally and Avoid Dangerous Orthopedic Surgery, Book/DVD, Whole Woman Inc., 2013

Katy Bowman, Dynamic Aging, Simple Exercises for Whole-Body Mobility, Propriometrics Press, 2017

Joseph M. Belanger, PT, Course presented by Manchester Community-Technical College, Manchester, CT, 1987

Dr. Steven Shifreen, Cranial-sacral therapy for brain trauma, eye glass adjustment, http://drshifreen.com/

Jill Peters-Gee, MD/Adine F. Fregan, MD, Training materials by Women's Health Specialty Care Urology, Urogynecology & Pelvic Health, Newington, CT, 2006

Personality/brain/inspirational:

Betty Edwards, Drawing on the Right Side of the Brain, J.P. Tracher, Inc, 1979; newer releases available

Tim LaHaye, Why You Act The Way You Do, Tyndale House Publishers, 1984 (owned several with other titles)

Mervyn Paul, Life-time is Training-time for Reigning Time, Truth & Tidings magazine, ~1975

Hannah Hurnard, Hinds' Feet on High Places, Tyndale House, 1977

Follow Others: Aging Wisdom from Beatitudes, Nature, Kinfolk

Norman Vincent Peale, The Power of Positive Thinking, Foundation for Christian Living, 1978

Joyce Meyer, Me and My Big Mouth! Your Answer is Right Under Your Nose, Harrison House, 1987

Dawna Markova, Ph.D, The Art of the Possible, A compassionate Approach to Understanding the Way People, Think, Learn & Communicate, Conari Press, 1991 (out of print)

Kevin Leman, The New Birth Order Book, Revell, revised 1998

Leslie Leyland Fields, Crossing the Waters: Following Jesus through the Storms, the Fish, the Doubt, and the Seas, NavPress, 2016

Daniel G. Amen, MD, Memory Rescue, Supercharge Your Brain, Reverse Memory loss, and Remember What Matters Most, Tyndale House Publishing, 2017

Dr. Caroline Leaf, Think Learn Succeed, Understanding and Using Your Mind to Thrive at School, the Workplace, and Life, Baker Books, 2018

Bekah DiFelice, Searching for Home in a Life on the Move, Nav Pres, 2018

Brian Hennings, Dancing in No Man's Land: Moving with Peace and Truth in a Hostile World, Nav Pres, 2018

The Great Courses – The Aging Brain DVD, Professor Thad A Polk, Ph.D. University of Michigan

Beauty:

Carole Jackson, Color Me Beautiful: Discover your natural beauty through the colors that make you look great, and feel fabulous,

Follow Others: Aging Wisdom from Beatitudes, Nature, Kinfolk

Ballantine Books, Revised 1987 (had earlier version) also, Color for Men, Ballantine Books, 1984

Andre Walker, Andre Talks Hair! (Special Message from Oprah Winfrey), Simon & Shuster, 1997

Lauren Cox with Janice Cox, Ecobeauty: Scrubs, Rubs, Masks, and Bath Bombs for You and Your Friends, Ten Speed Press, 2009

Financial:

Napoleon Hill, Think and Grow Rich, Penguin Group, 2005 (had older version)

Robert Kawasaki, Rich Dad, Poor Dad, What The Rich Teach Their Kids About Money That The Poor And Middle Class Do Not!, Plata Publishing, 2015 (had older version)

Suzie Orman, The 9 Steps to Financial Freedom: Practical and Spiritual Steps So You Can Stop Worrying, Random House, 1999

Other References/Quotes:

Saturday Evening Post, Nov/Dec, 2018

Follow Others: Aging Wisdom from Beatitudes, Nature, Kinfolk

[7 Tables; Entry-Chapter-page]

Indexes

—Aging Body—

Back—7-100, 8-113,117,118, 121, 12-193,195, 14-236

Brain—7-103, 10-147, 12-186,192,193

Dental—7-103to105

Ears—7-102

Eyes—7-98to102

Fat—7-97, 9-127,135,137, 10-156, 11-162,166

Female—9-127to134

Glands/Hormones—11-166,167,172, 12-188

Hair—6-67, 7-85to88, 9-135

Hemorrhoids/Colon—9-130

Hips—6-67,73, 8-114to118, 121, 12-182,186

Joints/Bones—8-113

Knees—8-113,116

Legs/Feet—7-97, 9-135, 11-172

Male—9-135to140

Nails—7-88

Neck—6-66, 75, 7-93, 8-115, 122, 12-182,186

Shoulder/Hand—7-96, 8-113, 116

Skin—6-66, 7-89to96, 9-125,144, 11-165, 12-182, 194,195

Ortho Tips:

Car—8-120,121

Chair—8-120,122

Mattress/Pillow—8-122,123

—Aging Issues/Diseases—

Arthritis—8-113

Autoimmune—6-67,68

Bladder—9-129,138,139

Blood—9-127,128

Bone Spurs—8-117

Brain—6-68to70,72

Follow Others: Aging Wisdom from Beatitudes, Nature, Kinfolk

Cancer—7-94to96, 7-110, 9-132,133,138,139

Cardio/ Heart—6-79, 12-183to185

Cholesterol—11-172,173

Diabetes—6-73, 7-95, 11-171,172

Falls—8-118

Gout—9-135,136,

Immunity—6-67

Indigestion—10-156to160

Kidney—9-136, 11-174,175,177,178

Liver—7-97, 11-173,174

Osteoporosis—8-115

Parkinson's—6-70, 12-182

Sleep—7-106

Smoking—12-186

Thyroid—6-71, 11-166,167

Urinary—9-130,138

Vaccines—7-107,108

—Diet/Therapy/Exercise—

Diets:

Blood Sugar—11-170to172

Blood Type—11-164to165

Body Type—11-166,167

Calories—11-167,168

Fasting—11-162,163,170

Fat-burning—11-169

Gluten—11-175,176

Hi-Low—11-168

Myths—11-161

Newest—11-162,169

Protein Drinks—11-178,179

Salt/Fluid—9-144, 11-176

Water—11-177

Therapy:

Heat vs. Cold—12-195

Massage—12-194

Naturopath—12-192

Ointments—12-194

Reflexology—AppA-256,257

Follow Others: Aging Wisdom from Beatitudes, Nature, Kinfolk

Exercise:

Body Type—12-186

CORE—12-181,189

Gender—12-187

Kegel—9-129, 138

Low-impact—12-188

Safety—12-189to190

Targeted—12-182

—Vitamins-Minerals/Herbs—

Generic—8-124

Female Issues—9-134

Male Issues—9-140

Supplements—6-63, 7-108

Probiotics—9-131, 10-159

Vitamins/Minerals:

Balance—9-142to145

Basics—6-67,76

Dr Shaklee—7-109,110

Guidelines—6-77, 7-84, 9-126

Youth restore—6-65, 79

Herbs:

Defense—AppA-255-257

Healers—14-238

Heart—9-143, 12-183to185

Overview—9-126, 14-238,239

Prostate—9-138,139

Spices—11-176,177, 14-238,239

Teas—10-149

—Homeopathy—

Arnica-injury—12-194, 14-239

Basics—5-61, 12-194,198to204

Cysts—7-96

Diarrhea—10-158

Defense—AppA-255to257

Female—9-134

FLU—7-107

Food poison—10-156

Ointments—12-194

Orthopedic—5-51, 13-215

Follow Others: Aging Wisdom from Beatitudes, Nature, Kinfolk

Pain Manage—8-118, 14-236to240

Remedies—12-192,199to202

Surgery—8-117

TMJ—7-105

Zinc—7-88,108, 9-139,143,144

—Mental Health/Styles—

Addictions/Habits—5-59

Depression/Anxiety—5-58,59

Forgiveness—5-56,62

Offenses—5-56

Relationship Rules—5-48, 49,51, 14-242,243

Singles—5-50,51, 14-234,242,243

Workplace—5-54,55

Victim/Bully—5-57

Positive Thinking:

Peale—4-42

Beatitudes—2-12

Apostles—4-40,41

Styles:

Communications—5-53,54

Financial—13-207to215

Temperaments—13-227to230

—Kinfolk—

Aunt Flossie—1-8

Uncle Ed—2-23, 14-242

Uncle Val—3-35

Letha—3- 35,14-247

Stone Masons—4-45

Edna—5-62

Nina—6-80

Dr. Shaklee—7-108

Achsa—9-141

Volunteers—10-155

My Kids—12-196

Flora G—13-225

Grandma F—14-247

Bert G—Afterword-251

Made in the USA
Middletown, DE
10 April 2021